UPPER EXTREMITY

INJURY EVALUATION CD AND ACTIVITY MANUAL

UPPER EXTREMITY
INJURY EVALUATION CD AND ACTIVITY MANUAL

Douglas Mann, DPE, ATC
Associate Professor
Health and Exercise Science Department
Rowan University
Glassboro, New Jersey

Colleen A. Grugan, MS, ATC, LAT
Assistant Athletic Trainer
Adjunct Professor, Health and Exercise Science Department
Rowan University
Glassboro, New Jersey

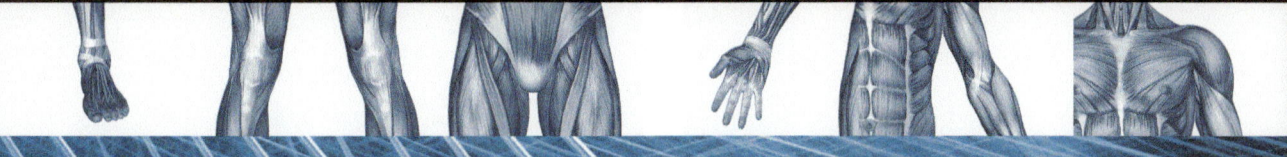

DELMAR
CENGAGE Learning

Australia • Brazil • Japan • Korea • Mexico • Singapore • Spain • United Kingdom • United States

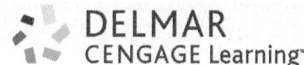
DELMAR
CENGAGE Learning™

Upper Extremity Injury Evaluation CD and Activity Manual
Douglas Mann and
Colleen A. Grugan

Vice President, Career and Professional Editorial: Dave Garza

Director of Learning Solutions: Matthew Kane

Acquisitions Editor: Matthew Seeley

Managing Editor: Marah Bellegarde

Product Manager: Jadin Babin-Kavanaugh

Editorial Assistant: Samantha Zullo

Vice President, Career and Professional Marketing: Jennifer Baker

Marketing Director: Wendy Mapstone

Marketing Manager: Kristin McNary

Marketing Coordinator: Erica Ropitzky

Production Director: Carolyn Miller

Production Manager: Andrew Crouth

Content Project Manager: Allyson Bozeth

Senior Art Director: Jack Pendleton

Technology Product Manager: Mary Colleen Liburdi

Technology Project Manager: Benjamin Knapp

Production Service: Pre-PressPMG

Library of Congress Control Number: 2009912990

ISBN-13: 978-1-4354-9925-6

ISBN-10: 1-4354-9925-5

Delmar
5 Maxwell Drive
Clifton Park, NY 12065-2919
USA

Cengage Learning is a leading provider of customized learning solutions with office locations around the globe, including Singapore, the United Kingdom, Australia, Mexico, Brazil, and Japan. Locate your local office at: **international.cengage.com/region**

Cengage Learning products are represented in Canada by Nelson Education, Ltd.

To learn more about Delmar, visit **www.cengage.com/delmar**

Purchase any of our products at your local college store or at our preferred online store **www.cengagebrain.com**

Printed in the United States of America
3 4 5 6 7   18 17 16 15

Table of Contents

Preface

This CD-ROM and activity manual offer you a visual aid to the systematic musculoskeletal evaluation process. It can be of benefit to virtually anyone seeking to learn more about the fields that perform orthopedic and/or musculoskeletal examinations—athletic training, physical therapy, and nursing, to name a few.

The CD program covers more parts of the evaluation process than any other resource on the market today, and engages users with the subject in a personal and adaptable way. This video and activity manual have been put together in a way that enables learners to retain by watching and practicing clinical skills rather than simply reading about them—pairing the power of video with student interaction and self-assessment will engage the user and enhance the overall learning experience. Performing self-evaluations will allow users to gain confidence and familiarity with the skills and knowledge they need to succeed both in the laboratory and in the real world. Additionally, the availability of video clips as skills for viewing "on the go" fits easily into any busy student's lifestyle.

ORGANIZATION OF THE *ACTIVITY MANUAL*

The *Activity Manual* is designed to enhance the video material and bridge the gap between classroom and homework by emphasizing practice and repetition of skills. The *Activity Manual* is divided into three sections, one for each body part covered. Each of those sections includes the following:

- **Landmark Identification:** Tests and/or refreshes knowledge of the location of the major anatomic landmarks.
- **Practical Examination:** Helps the learner prepare for future testing on clinical skills.
- **Scavenger Hunt:** A creative and fun way to view and review the evaluation skills video content on the CD.
- **Peer Assessment:** Similar to the practical examinations, each peer assessment can be used to provide a first assessment to clinical evaluations and for the learner to reflect on their readiness for professional evaluation.
- **Special Test Sub-Skills:** Require the learner to think about the skills necessary to perform any special and/or ligamentous tests.
- **Related Questions:** Test knowledge about the body part being evaluated.
- **Palpation Lesson:** Helps the learner think about anatomic landmarks and how to establish their location.

Section IV is the directed **Observation Assignment**, designed to encourage the user to get an experience and ask questions during this experience.

ALSO AVAILABLE-ONLINE COMPANION RESOURCE SITE

Video-on-demand applications for iTouch and iPod are available for download at iTunes. For more information and additional resources, go to www.delmarlearning.com/companions. In the search field in the upper right corner, enter 'Mann' as the search term, then click on the link for this book.

ABOUT THE AUTHORS

Douglas Mann, DPE, ATC

Rowan University, Glassboro, New Jersey

Douglas Mann earned his undergraduate degree from University of Miami (Fla), his Master's degree from Old Dominion University, and his Doctorate from Springfield College. He has worked as an athletic trainer at the high school, college, olympic trial, and professional levels. He is currently an associate professor in Health and Exercise Science at Rowan University.

Colleen A. Grugan, MS, ATC

Rowan University, Glassboro, New Jersey

Colleen Grugan received her undergraduate degree from Rowan University (NJ), and her Master's degree from Georgia Southern University. She has worked at the high school and college levels. Colleen currently serves as the assistant athletic trainer at her alma mater, Rowan University. She also serves as an adjunct professor in Rowan's Health and Exercise Science Department, teaching several of the Athletic Training Education laboratories.

REVIEWERS

Special thanks are extended by the authors and publisher to the reviewers who provided recommendations and suggestions to improve this product every step of the way. Their experience and knowledge has been a valuable resource.

Art Bartolozzi, MD

Chief of Sports Medicine, Pennsylvania Hospital

Associate Clinical Professor of Orthopaedic Surgery, University of Pennsylvania

Team Physician, Rowan University

Dr. Diane Bartholomew, ATC

Associate Professor and Chair

Division of Health and Movement Science

Athletic Training Curriculum Director

Graceland University

Lamoni, Iowa

David C. Berry, PhD, ATC, EMT-B

Assistant Professor, Coordinator of Clinical Education and Athletic Therapy Program Director

Weber State University

Ogden, Utah

Barbara Blackstone, MSS, ATC, LAT

Assistant Professor, Coordinator of Athletic Training Education

University of Maine—Presque Isle

Presque Isle, Maine

Jennifer Jordan Hamson-Utley, PhD, LAT, ATC

Assistant Professor, ATEP Program Director

Weber State University

Ogden, Utah

Timothy G. Howell, EdD, ATC, CSCS

Athletic Training Education Program Director

Alfred University

Alfred, New York

William T. Lyons, MS, ATC

Athletic Training Program Director

Division of Kinesiology

University of Wyoming

Laramie, Wyoming

Sharon Menegoni, MS, ATC

Assistant Professor and Program Director of Athletic Training

Longwood University

Farmville, Virginia

Julie A. Snyder, MS Ed, ACE CPT

Program Director

Sports Medicine & Fitness Technology

Keiser University

Port St. Lucie, Florida

Adam Thompson, PhD

Director of Athletic Training Education

Indiana Wesleyan University

Marion, Indiana

ACKNOWLEDGMENTS

I would like to thank the athletic training education students at Rowan University, especially those who assisted with this project. In addition, I would like to thank my colleagues at Rowan University who I have the immense pleasure of working with. I also very much need to thank Rhonda Fabian and Jerry Baber, and their staff, who were competent, professional, and made the CD so much better. My thanks also go to Delmar, especially Matt and

Jadin for believing in this project and supporting it all the way. Many thanks to my wife, Neeli, who adopted this project with me. Lastly, I wish to thank my children, AJ and Addi, who give me more happiness than I ever thought possible.

Doug Mann

I want to first thank Delmar, especially Jadin and Matt. Without them, this project would never have been possible. Many thanks need to go to Rhonda Fabian and Jerry Baber, along with their staff, for helping to make this project unique and for being very understanding throughout the process. To Doug Mann—thank you for including me in this project, and for being a huge part of the professional I am today. Thank you to the Rowan University Athletic Training Education students who helped with this project and volunteered their time and thoughts. Thanks to Chuck Whedon, MS, ATC for all his support and wisdom, and to David Heim, MS, ATC for letting me pick his brain and use his camera. Thanks to Christina Ludlam, ATC for ideas and for being a rock. And most of all, to my parents—you push me to be better, but love me no matter what. Thanks!

Colleen A. Grugan

TO THE LEARNER: HOW TO USE THE *INJURY EVALUATION CD* AND *ACTIVITY MANUAL*

This interactive CD-ROM and activity manual is designed to provide you with the means to review comprehensive demonstrations of the clinical skills associated with an orthopedic evaluation. It can be difficult to read about hands-on skills and to fully interpret the required movements from a still photograph or illustration. This video program allows you to view a clinical skill in its entirety, and to complete a self-evaluation on the subject area you're working in, as many times as you like. While watching the video program is certainly no substitute for hands-on skills practice, a confident understanding of when and why these skills are performed is essential for a complete and accurate assessment. For more about how to use the video program, see next section "How to Use the Interactive Video Program."

For more independent learning, the activity manual can be used to enhance your understanding of orthopedic clinical evaluation skills. For example, the Practical Examinations are similar to those examinations used in our evaluation classes, and can help provide you with feedback on your ability to perform a clinical evaluation and reach an accurate diagnosis. The practical examinations will help develop and increase your competence and comfort level in performing orthopedic evaluations.

The Peer Assessments, while not comprehensive, can also serve as a study guide, and encourage you to practice skills with your peers.

The Scavenger Hunt was designed as a creative way for the student to make use of the interactive Video program. The Special Tests and Palpation activities are an opportunity for you to begin to think about how to teach the skills associated with the orthopedic evaluation. At the conclusion of the activity manual is an assignment based on observing orthopedic evaluations. This assignment is meant to help direct you during an observation experience in a lab, athletic training room, or other facility.

TO THE LEARNER: HOW TO USE THE INTERACTIVE VIDEO PROGRAM

The interactive program on the CD-ROM is designed to help you review and assess your knowledge of the skills covered. Use the program as your own private tutorial to help you review and practice the material covered in regular lectures. You must have access to either a PC or MAC computer with a CD-ROM or a DVD-ROM drive to utilize this interactive program.

MAIN MENU

From the Main Menu, you may choose one of three subject areas to study, or choose to take the comprehensive Test. It is recommended that you take the comprehensive Test after completing each subject area.

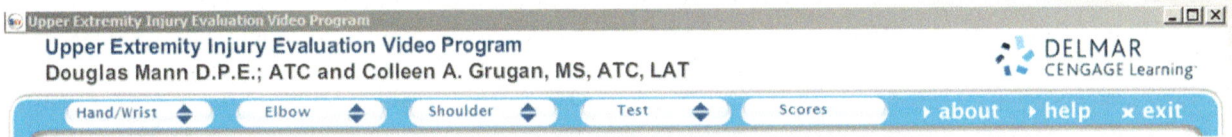

SUBJECT AREAS

When you click on a particular subject area from the Main Menu, you will see a branching menu that includes videos and a Self-Assessment.

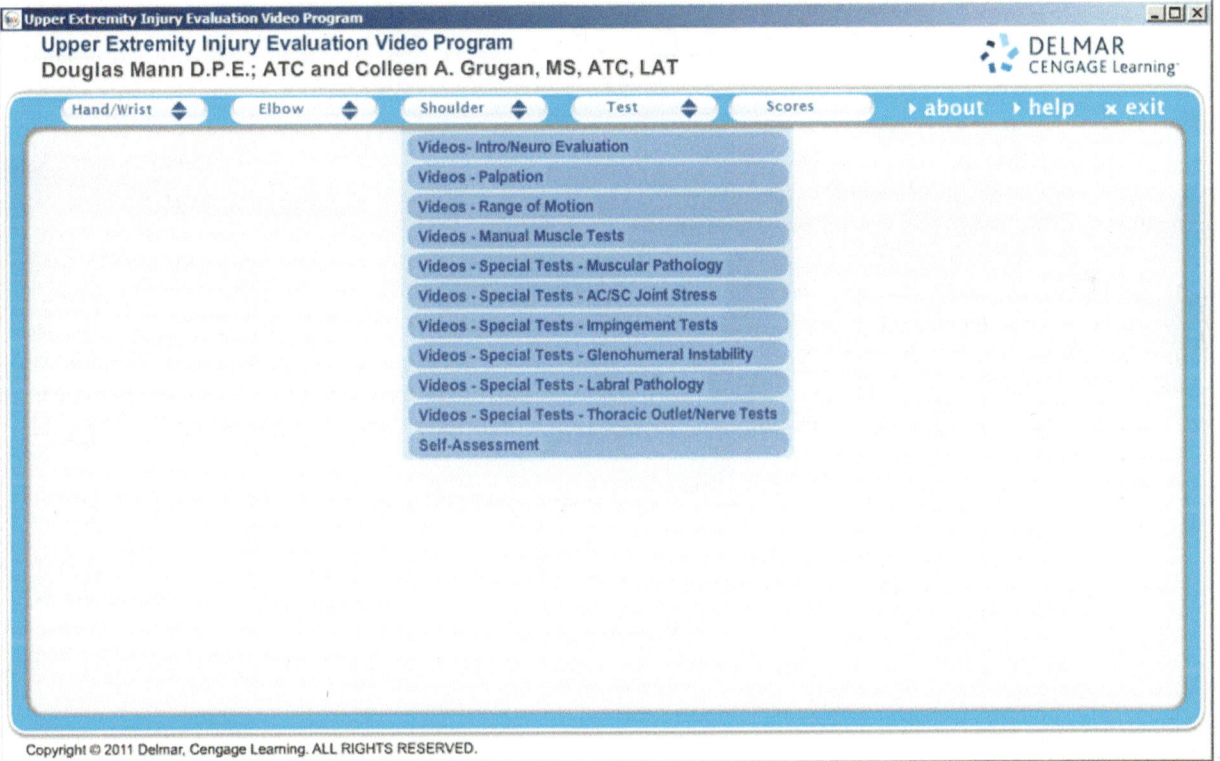

SELF-ASSESSMENTS

Within each subject area, you will notice a Self-Assessment tab on the menu. This is a randomized quiz that provides you with immediate right and wrong answer feedback, allowing you to self-test and review as you proceed. The Self-Assessment module includes the following question types: multiple choice, matching, fill-in-the-blank, and image labeling exercises. Some questions may require you to view a video or read a scenario in order to answer the question.

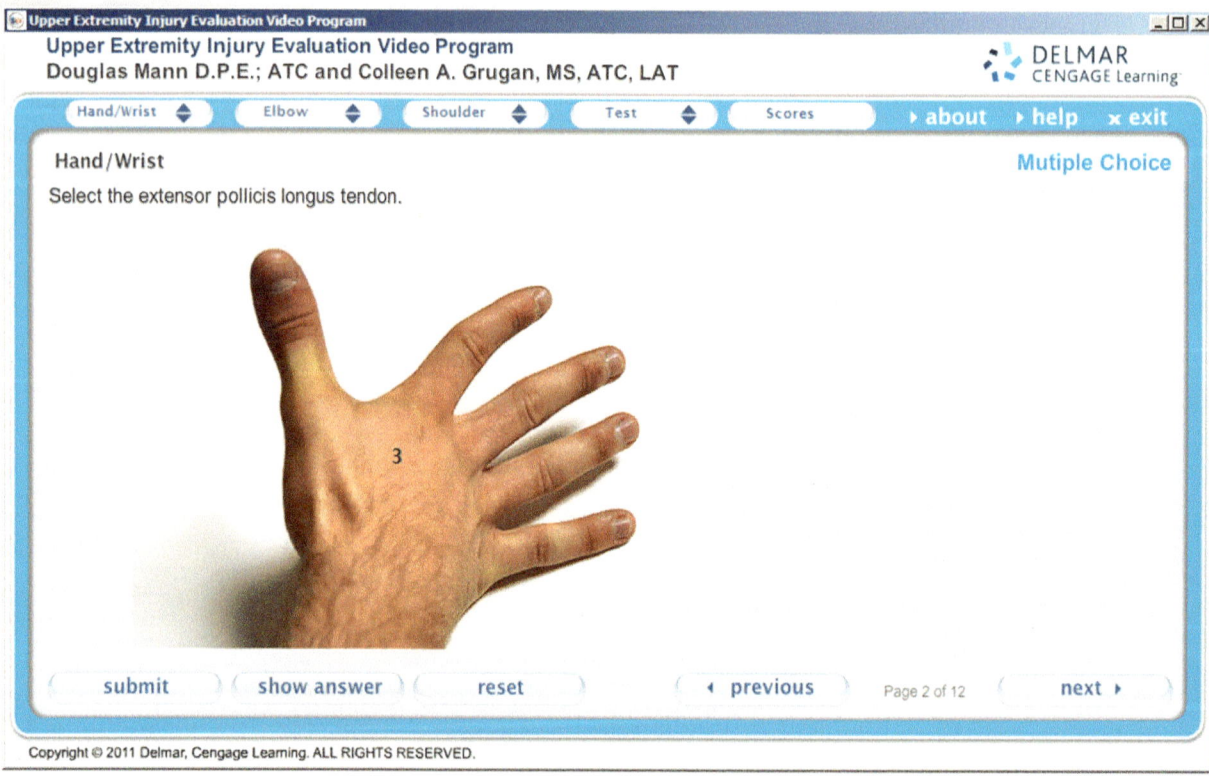

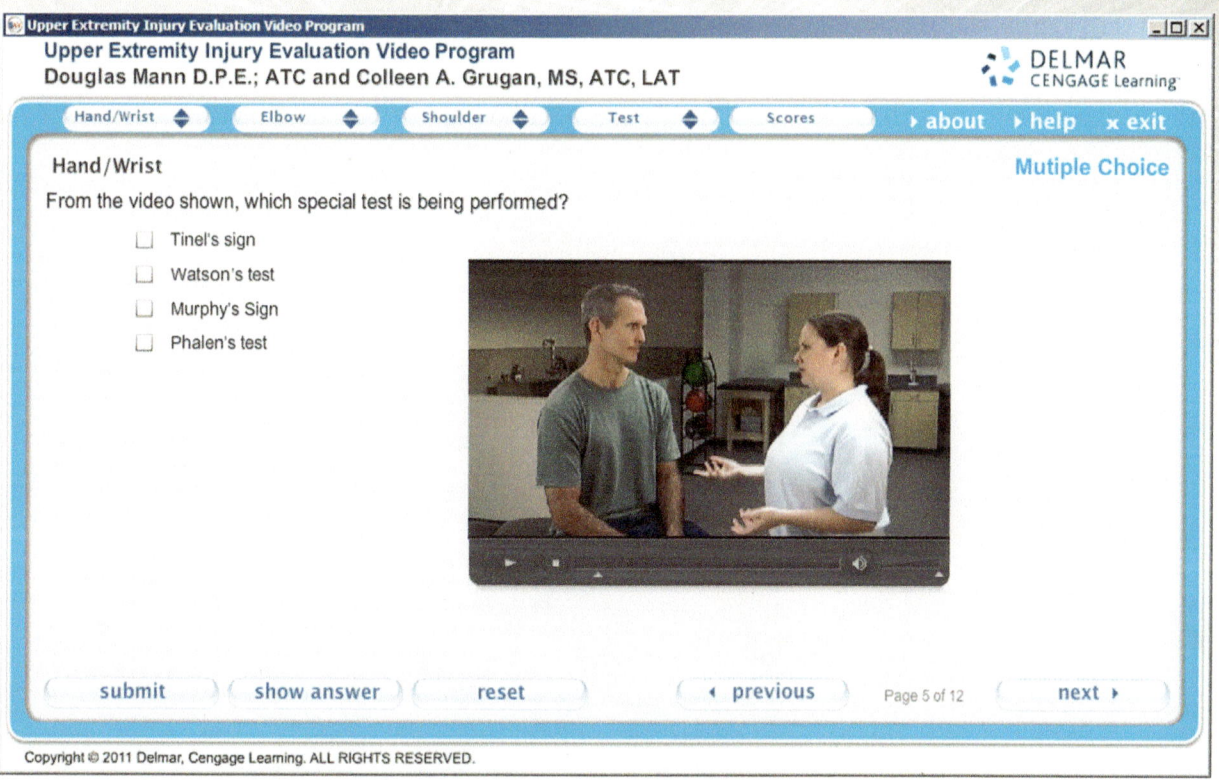

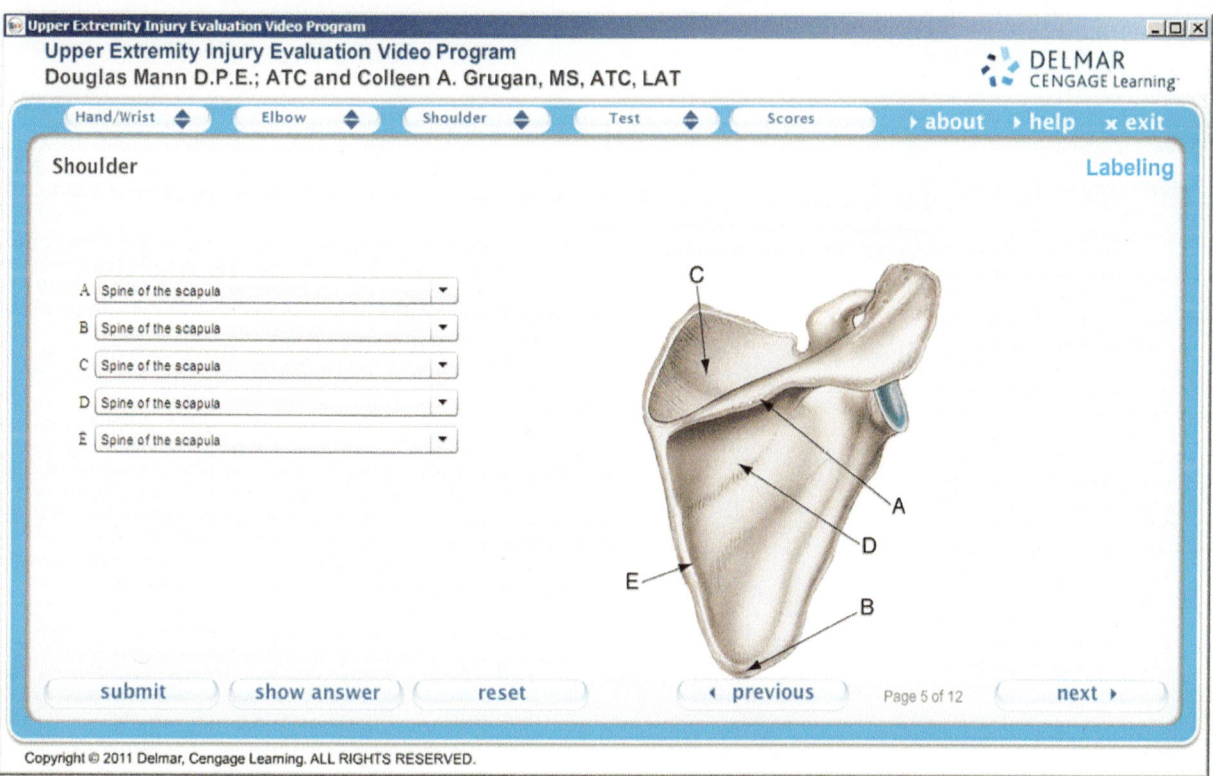

VIDEOS

The videos are listed under four headings: Palpation, Range of Motion, Manual Muscle Tests, and Special Tests. View one video at a time by clicking on each. Go to the next set of videos by clicking the Next button.

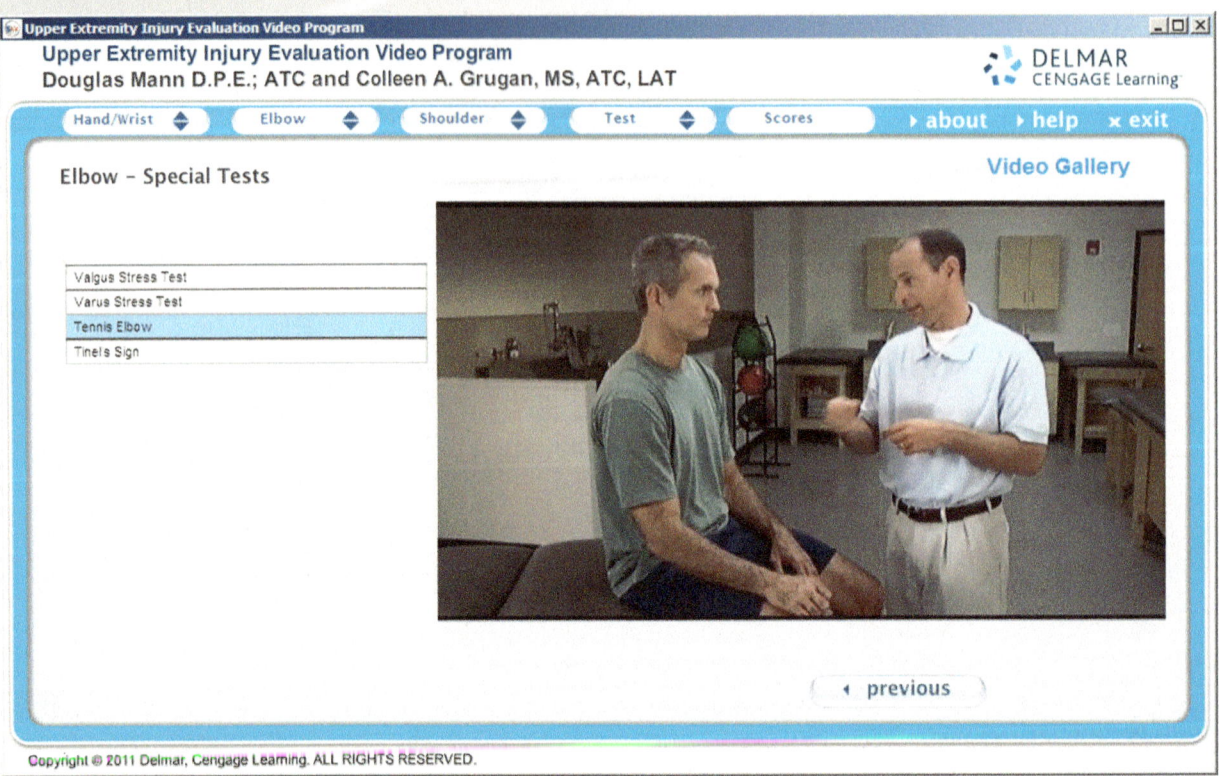

COMPREHENSIVE TEST

The test tab on the Main Menu screen will take you to a comprehensive test that covers all three subject areas covered on the CD. Take this test after you have been through each module and have completed the self-assessment in each. Your scores will be recorded when you take the comprehensive test, and can be printed out and handed in as directed by your instructor.

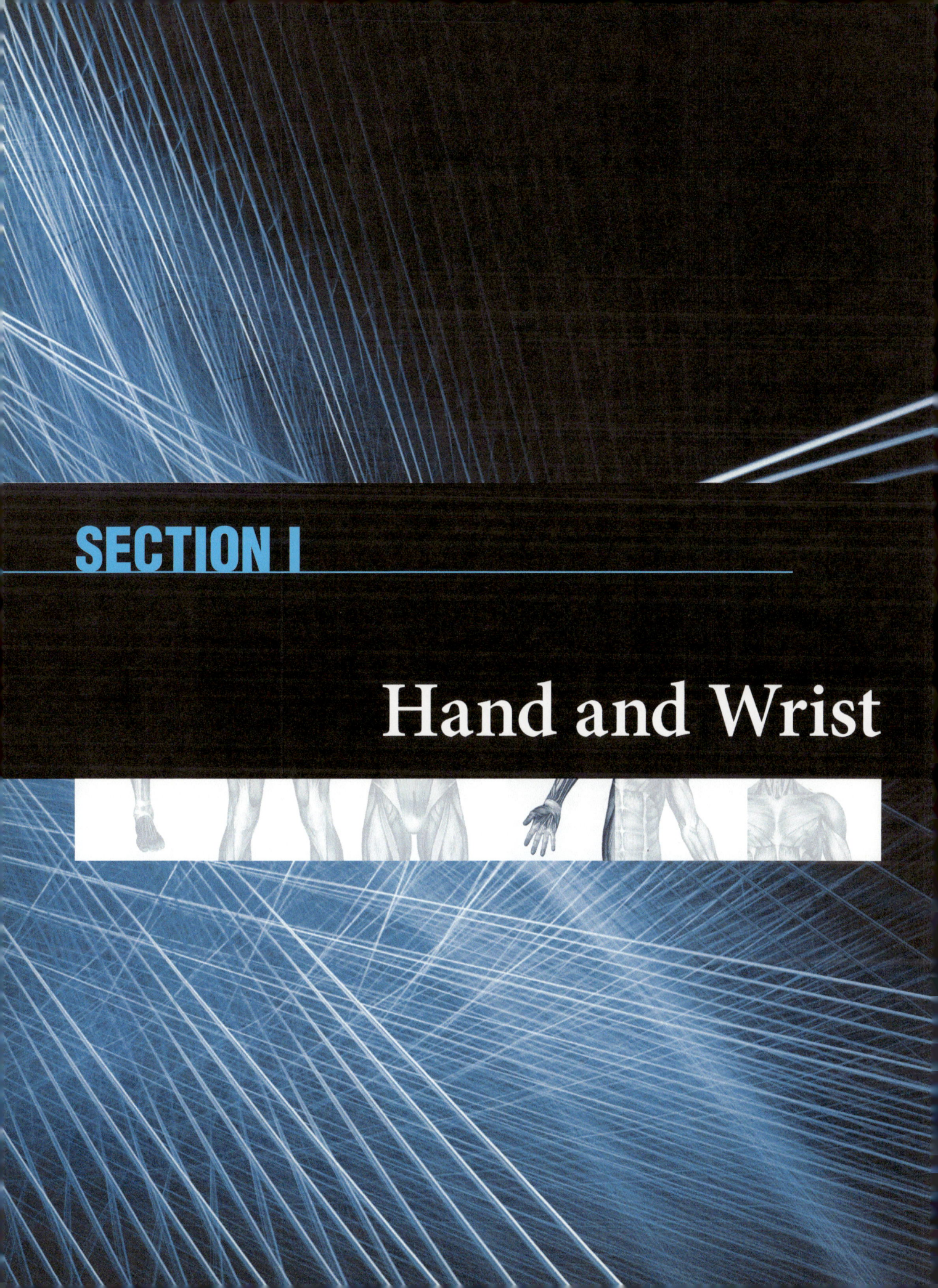

SECTION I

Hand and Wrist

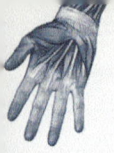

HAND AND WRIST

LANDMARK IDENTIFICATION

Identify the structures in Figures 1-1 through 1-3. Consult a medical atlas as needed.

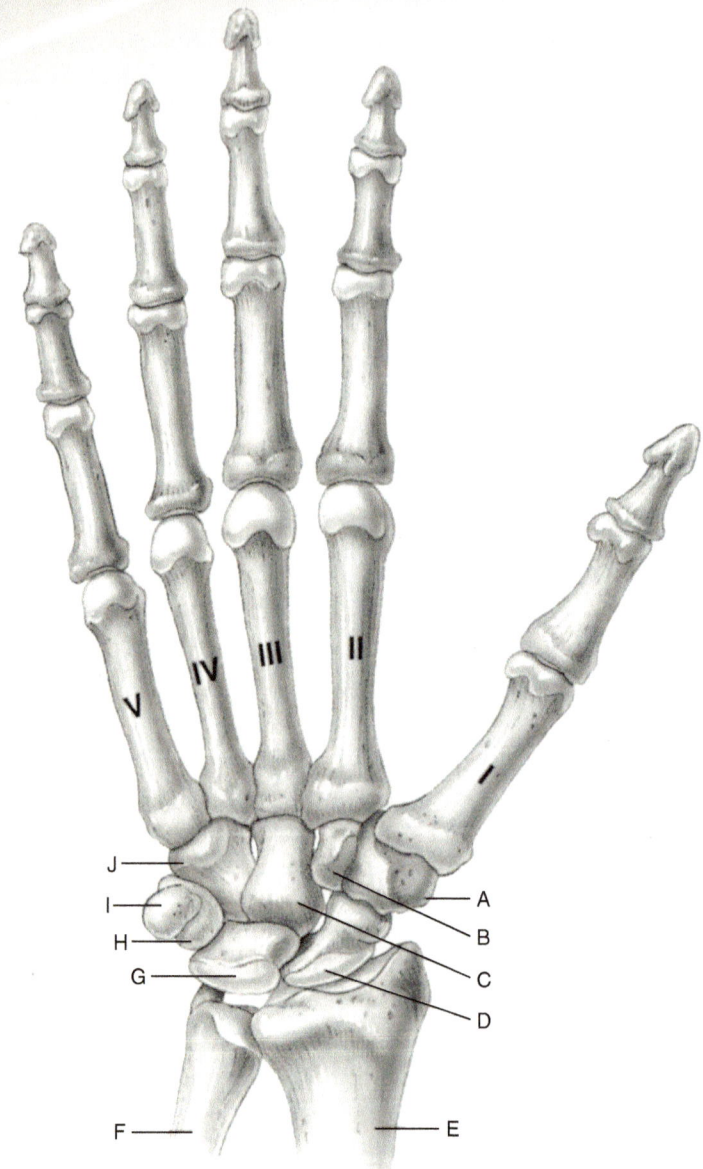

FIGURE 1-1

A. _____ F. _____
B. _____ G. _____
C. _____ H. _____
D. _____ I. _____
E. _____ J. _____

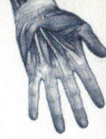

Anterior View

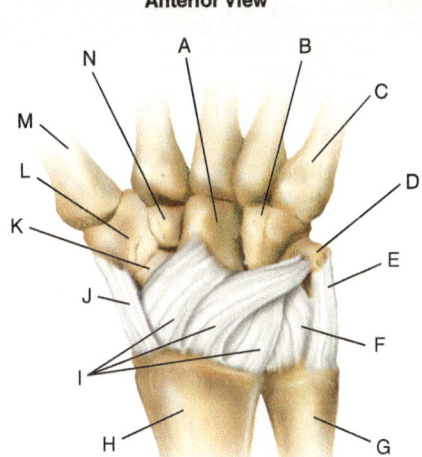

Posterior View

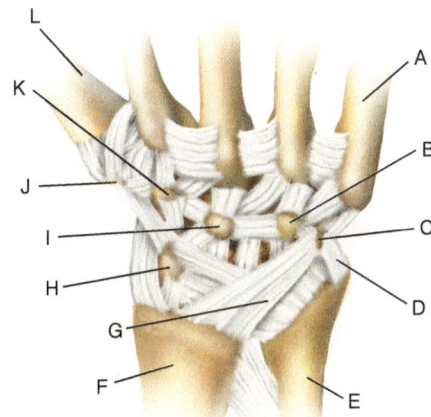

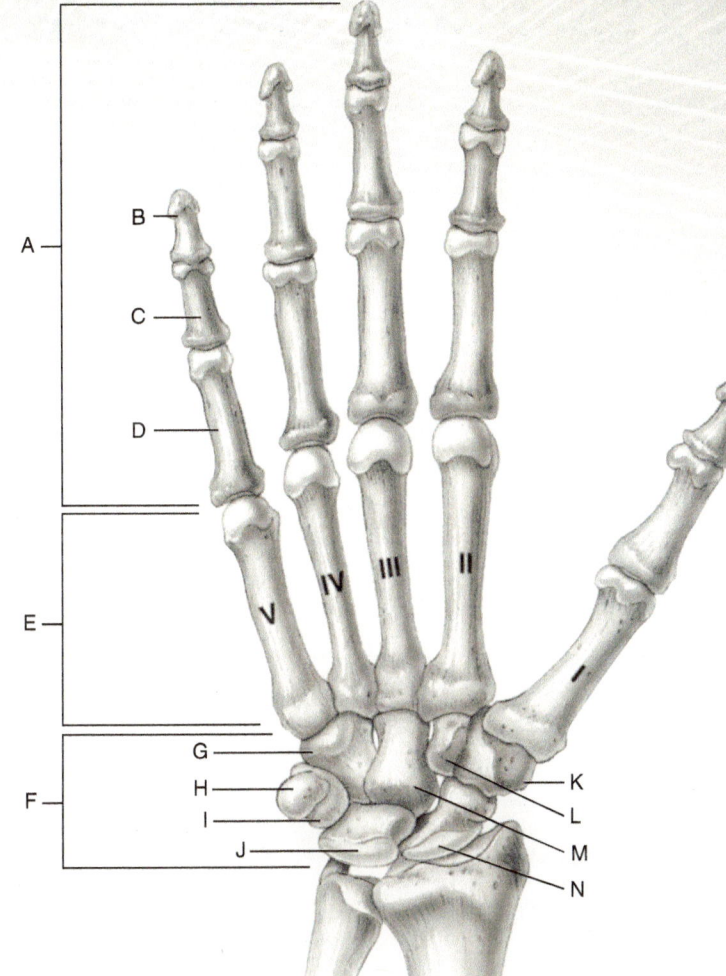

FIGURE 1-2

Anterior View

A. _____ H. _____
B. _____ I. _____
C. _____ J. _____
D. _____ K. _____
E. _____ L. _____
F. _____ M. _____
G. _____ N. _____

Posterior View

A. _____ H. _____
B. _____ I. _____
C. _____ J. _____
D. _____ K. _____
E. _____ L. _____
F. _____
G. _____

FIGURE 1-3

A. _____ H. _____
B. _____ I. _____
C. _____ J. _____
D. _____ K. _____
E. _____ L. _____
F. _____ M. _____
G. _____ N. _____

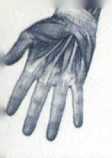

HAND AND WRIST

 # PRACTICAL EXAMINATIONS

Directions: Have another student or professional administer these oral practical examinations. The administrator will read through each list, watch as you perform each task, and mark as you complete it. The person administering the examination should read only the numbered instructions.

PRACTICAL EXAMINATION 1

1. A patient hurt his wrist in a game two weeks ago. It has gotten progressively worse and now he is seeking an evaluation from a medical professional. Complete a history for the injury.

QUESTIONS TO ASK PATIENT	COMPLETED (Y/N)/COMMENTS
Where is the pain?	
What kind of pain (for example, numbness, or tingling) are you experiencing?	
What level of pain (from 1 to 10, with 10 being the worst) are you experiencing?	
Are there any movements or activities that make the pain worse, or better?	
What is the mechanism of the injury?	
How did the injury occur?	
When the injury occurred, did you hear any sounds?	
Were you able to keep playing on the injury?	
Have you done or had any treatment for the injury?	
Have you had an injury like this in the past?	
Other pertinent history questions	

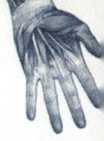

2. You are now ready to complete the observation phase of the evaluation. Perform the observation portion of your evaluation, assuming you did not see this individual walk in.

ACTIONS	COMPLETED (Y/N)/COMMENTS
Observe how the patient is carrying the injured hand/wrist	
Check injured area for swelling	
Check injured area for deformity	
Check injured area for discoloration	
Perform bilateral comparison	
Check muscle tone	
Check skin temperature of injured area	
Check facial expression for pain	
Other pertinent observations	

3. Palpate the following anatomical landmarks.

PALPATION	COMPLETED (Y/N)/COMMENTS
Scaphoid	
Ulnar styloid process	
Palmaris longus	
Flexor carpi radialis	
Extensor pollicis longus tendon	
Capitate	

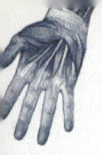

HAND AND WRIST

4. Perform the following range of motion tests. (The administrator should mark if each component was done.) Skills should be performed by the examiner unless otherwise noted.

A. Passive Range of Motion for Wrist Flexion

	COMPLETED (Y/N)/COMMENTS
Brings patient's wrist into flexion	
Stabilizes patient's wrist	
Performs test bilaterally	

B. Resistive Range of Motion for Wrist Extension

	COMPLETED (Y/N)/COMMENTS
Provides resistance as patient moves through wrist extension	
Stabilizes patient's wrist	
Performs test bilaterally	

C. Goniometric Test for Wrist Extension

	COMPLETED (Y/N)/COMMENTS
Places fulcrum on triquetrum	
Aligns movement arm with fifth metacarpal	
Aligns stationary arm with ulna	
Measures correctly	

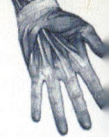

5. Perform the following manual muscle tests. The administrator will check each item as you complete it. Skills should be performed by the examiner unless otherwise noted.

A. Flexor Digitorum Profundus

	COMPLETED (Y/N)/COMMENTS
Stabilizes patient's proximal and middle phalanges	
Resists flexion of the dip joint	
Performs test bilaterally	
Performs isometric break test	

B. Abductor Pollicis Longus

	COMPLETED (Y/N)/COMMENTS
Stabilizes patient's wrist	
Resists thumb abduction	
Performs test bilaterally	
Performs isometric break test	

C. Flexor Digitorum Superficialis

	COMPLETED (Y/N)/COMMENTS
Stabilizes the patient's metacarpophalangeal (MCP) joint	
Resists flexion of the pip joint	
Performs test bilaterally	
Performs isometric break test	

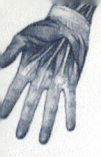

6. Perform the following ligamentous/special tests. The administrator will check each item as you complete it. Skills should be performed by the examiner unless otherwise noted.

   A. Watson's Test

	COMPLETED (Y/N)/COMMENTS
Has patient seated or standing	
Grips patient's scaphoid bone	
Applies gliding motion in anterior/posterior directions	
Adds radial/ulnar deviation if no pain present	
Understands purpose of Watson's test and what constitutes a positive test	

   B. Phalen's Test

	COMPLETED (Y/N)/COMMENTS
Has patient seated or standing	
Has patient with back of hands in contact	
Has patient with both wrists in full flexion	
Has patient hold position for one minute	
Understands purpose of Phalen's test and what constitutes a positive test	

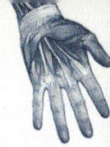

C. Murphy's Sign

	COMPLETED (Y/N)/COMMENTS
Instructs patient to make a fist	
Observes patient's third metacarpal	
Performs test bilaterally	
Understands purpose of Murphy's sign test and what constitutes a positive test	

D. Finkelstein's Test

	COMPLETED (Y/N)/COMMENTS
Instructs patient to make a fist with thumb tucked inside	
Passively ulnar deviates patient's wrist	
Stabilizes patient's forearm	
Performs test bilaterally	
Understands purpose of Finkelstein's test and what constitutes a positive test	

7. Perform a dermatome test for the upper extremity. The administrator will check each item as you complete it.

	COMPLETED (Y/N)/COMMENTS
C1 (Top of head)	
C2 (side of face, temple area)	
C3 (angle of mandible)	
C4 (side of neck)	
C5 (proximal lateral arm, deltoid area)	
C6 (lateral forearm, thumb)	
C7 (middle forearm, 3rd finger)	
C8 (medial forearm, 5th finger)	
T1 (medial humerus)	

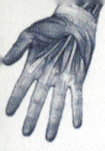

PRACTICAL EXAMINATION 2

1. A field hockey player comes into your athletic training room complaining of wrist pain that she has been experiencing for one month. She is now seeking an evaluation from a medical professional. Complete a history for the injury.

QUESTIONS TO ASK PATIENT	COMPLETED (Y/N)/COMMENTS
Where is the pain?	
What kind of pain (for example, numbness, or tingling) are you experiencing?	
What level of pain (from 1 to 10, with 10 being the worst) are you experiencing?	
Are there any movements or activities that make the pain worse, or better?	
What is the mechanism of the injury?	
How did the injury occur?	
When the injury occurred, did you hear any sounds?	
Were you able to keep playing on the injury?	
Have you done or had any treatment for the injury?	
Have you had an injury like this in the past?	
Other pertinent history questions	

2. You are now ready to complete the observation phase of the evaluation. Perform the observation portion of your evaluation, assuming you did not see this individual walk in.

ACTIONS	COMPLETED (Y/N)/COMMENTS
Observe how the patient is carrying the injured hand/wrist	
Check injured area for swelling	
Check injured area for deformity	
Check injured area for discoloration	
Perform bilateral comparison	
Check muscle tone	
Check skin temperature of injured area	
Check facial expression for pain	
Other pertinent observations	

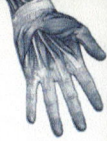

3. Palpate the following anatomical landmarks.

PALPATION	COMPLETED (Y/N)/COMMENTS
Lunate	
Thenar eminence	
Triangular fibrocartilage complex (TFCC)	
Radial artery	
Extensor pollicis longus	
Ulnar collateral ligament of the thumb	

4. Perform the following range of motion tests. (The administrator should mark if each component was done.) Skills should be performed by the examiner unless otherwise noted.

   A. Passive Range of Motion for Wrist Extension

	COMPLETED (Y/N)/COMMENTS
Brings patient's wrist into extension	
Stabilizes patient's wrist	
Performs test bilaterally	

   B. Resistive Range of Motion for Wrist Flexion

	COMPLETED (Y/N)/COMMENTS
Provides resistance as patient moves through wrist flexion	
Stabilizes patient's wrist	
Performs test bilaterally	

   C. Goniometric Test for Ulnar Deviation

	COMPLETED (Y/N)/COMMENTS
Places fulcrum on capitate	
Aligns movement arm with third metacarpal	
Aligns stationary arm with midline of forearm	
Measures correctly	

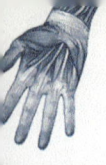

5. Perform the following manual muscle tests. The administrator will check each item as you complete it. Skills should be performed by the examiner unless otherwise noted.

A. Extensor Pollicis Longus

	COMPLETED (Y/N)/COMMENTS
Stabilizes patient's wrist	
Resists thumb extension	
Performs test bilaterally	
Performs isometric break test	

B. Adductor Pollicis

	COMPLETED (Y/N)/COMMENTS
Stabilizes patient's wrist	
Resists thumb adduction	
Performs test bilaterally	
Performs isometric break test	

C. Flexor Digitorum Superficialis

	COMPLETED (Y/N)/COMMENTS
Stabilizes the patient's MCP joint	
Resists flexion of the pip joint	
Performs test bilaterally	
Performs isometric break test	

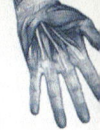

6. Perform the following ligamentous/special tests. The administrator will check each item as you complete it. Skills should be performed by the examiner unless otherwise noted.

A. Grip Test

	COMPLETED (Y/N)/COMMENTS
Has patient seated or standing	
Instructs patient to squeeze examiner's hand	
Compares strength bilaterally	
Understands purpose of grip test and what constitutes a positive test	

B. Digital Allen Test

	COMPLETED (Y/N)/COMMENTS
Asks patient to open and close hand several times	
Has patient make a fist	
Compresses patient's radial and ulnar artery	
Releases pressure one artery at a time	
Understands purpose of digital Allen test and what constitutes a positive test	

C. Murphy's Sign

	COMPLETED (Y/N)/COMMENTS
Instructs patient to make a fist	
Observes patient's third metacarpal	
Performs test bilaterally	
Understands purpose of Murphy's sign test and what constitutes a positive test	

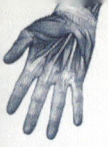

D. Froment's Sign

	COMPLETED (Y/N)/COMMENTS
Instructs patient to hold a piece of paper between thumb and index finger	
Attempts to pull paper away from patient	
Understands purpose of Froment's sign and what constitutes a positive test	

7. **Perform** a myotome test for the upper extremity. The administrator will check each item as you complete it.

	COMPLETED (Y/N)/COMMENTS
C1 (neck flexion)	
C2 (neck flexion)	
C3 (neck lateral flexion)	
C4 (shoulder elevation)	
C5 (shoulder abduction)	
C6 (elbow flexion, wrist extension)	
C7 (elbow extension, wrist flexion)	
C8 (thumb extension, ulnar deviation)	
T1 (finger abduction, adduction)	

 ## SCAVENGER HUNT

Read the following questions and try to find the answers by watching the CD enclosed with this text.

1. What palpation is described as the last bone in the proximal row for the carpals?

_____

_____

2. What palpation is described as the largest of the carpal bones?

_____

_____

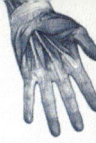

3. What two tendons form the radial border of the anatomic snuff box?

_____

_____

4. What is the mechanism of injury mentioned in the palpation section for TFCC pathology?

_____

_____

5. What is considered the normal goniometric measurement for ulnar deviation?

_____

_____

6. What joint do you stabilize when testing the flexor digitorum superficialis?

_____

_____

7. According to the CD, what muscles are tested during the grip test?

_____

_____

8. What is considered a positive test for the carpal glide test?

_____

_____

9. How long is Phalen's test held?

_____

_____

10. What is Murphy's sign?

_____

_____

 ## PEER ASSESSMENTS

Ask a fellow classmate or peer to assess your performance of the following evaluation procedures. After the peer assessment is completed, answer the post-assessment questions on your own. When you feel confident in your proficiency, you may want to re-test your performance of these skills with a professional acting as your peer reviewer.

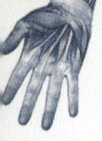

HAND AND WRIST

PEER ASSESSMENT 1

EVALUATION SKILLS	DATE OF ASSESSMENT	CORRECT/NOT CORRECT	COMMENTS
Palpations Lister's tubercle Radial styloid process Pisiform Lunate Scaphoid			
Range of Motion Active wrist extension Passive ulnar deviation Goniometric measurement wrist flexion			
Manual Muscle Tests Adductor pollicis Flexor digitorum superficialis Extensor pollicis longus			
Ligamentous/Special Tests Tinel's sign Froment's sign Murphy's sign			
Neurological Tests Dermatome assessment upper extremity C1–T8			
Reviewer's Signature: _____ Date: _____			

Post-Assessment Questions

1. Did you feel confident during the peer assessment?

   _____

   _____

2. Which skills (manual muscle tests, range of motion, etc.) did you feel most confident completing, and why?

   _____

   _____

3. Which skill did you feel least confident completing, and why?

   _____

   _____

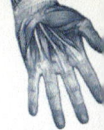

PEER ASSESSMENT 2

Perform this assessment at least two weeks after completing Peer Assessment 1. Follow the directions provided for the first peer assessment.

EVALUATION SKILLS	DATE OF ASSESSMENT	CORRECT/NOT CORRECT	COMMENTS
Palpations Thenar eminence Pisiform Hook of hamate Extensor pollicis longus			
Range of Motion Active finger flexion Passive radial deviation Goniometric wrist extension			
Manual Muscle Tests Flexor digitorum profundis Flexor pollicis longus Abductor pollicis brevis			
Ligamentous/Special Tests Lunatotriquetral (Reagan's) Bunnel littler Long finger flexor			
Neurological Tests Myotome testing C1–T8			
Reviewer's Signature: _____		Date: _____	

Post-Assessment Questions

1. Do you feel more comfortable with the evaluation of the hand and wrist than you did during the first assessment? Why or why not?

    _____

    _____

2. In which area (manual muscle tests, special tests, etc.) do you have the most confidence in your abilities, and why?

    _____

    _____

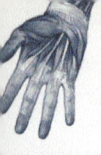

3. In which area do you feel the least confident in your abilities, and why?

    _____

    _____

4. Name three palpations of the hand and wrist that you have no difficulty locating. (Note: these do not need to be palpations discussed in this assessment.)

    _____

    _____

5. Name three palpations of the hand and wrist that tend to be challenging for you to find. (Note: these do not need to be palpations discussed in this assessment.)

    _____

    _____

PEER ASSESSMENT 3

Perform this assessment at least two weeks after completing Peer Assessment 2. This assessment should take longer than Assessments 1 and 2. Ask a fellow classmate or peer to develop their own questions in the following categories and assess your performance. After the peer assessment is completed, answer the post-assessment questions on your own. When you feel confident with your proficiency, you may want to re-test your performance of these skills with a professional acting as your peer reviewer.

EVALUATION SKILLS	DATE OF ASSESSMENT	CORRECT/NOT CORRECT	COMMENTS
Palpations of the hand and wrist			
Range of motion of the hand and wrist			
Manual muscle tests of the hand and wrist			
Ligamentous/special tests of the hand and wrist			
Neurological tests of the hand and wrist (dermatomes, myotomes, and reflexes)			
Reviewer's Signature: _____			Date: _____

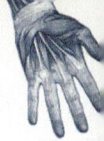

Post-Assessment Questions

1. Do you feel competent in performing an evaluation of the hand and wrist in order to reach a diagnosis?

    _____

    _____

2. With regards to the hand and wrist, what do you feel is the most important part of the injury evaluation process, and why?

    _____

    _____

3. How have your evaluation skills improved from the first assessment to the third?

    _____

    _____

4. How can you continue to improve your evaluation skills?

    _____

    _____

SPECIAL TEST SUB-SKILLS

For the special tests listed, write out the sub-skills necessary for skill completion. In addition, list what each special test is for and what constitutes a positive test. The first one has been done for you as an example.

TEST	SUB-SKILLS	STRUCTURE(S) TESTED	POSITIVE TEST INDICATION
Phalen's	• *Has the patient seated or standing* • *Has patient hold both wrists maximally flexed with back of hands touching* • *Has patient hold position for one minute*	*This test checks for carpal tunnel syndrome (median nerve compression).*	*A positive test is indicated by numbness, tingling, or pain along the median nerve.*
Watson's			
Long finger flexor			
Bunnel littler			

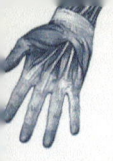

HAND AND WRIST

Complete the below exercise for four additional special or ligament tests.

TEST	SUB-SKILLS	STRUCTURE(S) TESTED	POSITIVE TEST INDICATION

RELATED HAND AND WRIST QUESTIONS

1. A benign mass (tumor) usually seen on the dorsal side of the wrist is referred to as a _____ cyst.

2. What structure is involved in the pathology Gamekeeper's Thumb?

   _____

   _____

3. What is the difference between "jersey finger" and "mallet finger"?

   _____

   _____

4. What is the most commonly fractured bone in the hand?

   _____

   _____

5. What is the most commonly dislocated bone in the wrist?

   _____

   _____

6. When measuring ulnar deviation the fulcrum is placed on the _____.

7. A disease that results in necrosis of the lunate bone due to a loss of blood supply is called _____.

8. Blood trapped under the fingernail is referred to as a _____.

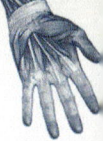

9. The two major nerves that innervate the wrist and hand are the _____ and _____.

10. Bringing the thumb and little finger together is an example of _____.

11. A fracture of the first metacarpal that extends into the articular surface is called a _____ fracture.

12. Fractures of the fifth metacarpal are termed _____ fractures.

13. When splinting a mallet finger, the distal interphalangeal (DIP) joint should be in _____.

14. There are _____ carpal bones in the hand.

15. Movement of the hand toward the radial side is termed _____.

16. Fill in the following chart for each muscle of the hand or wrist. The first one has been done for you as an example.

MUSCLE	ORIGIN	INSERTION	ACTION	INNERVATION
Flexor digitorum profundis	Upper 3/4 of ulna, medial epicondyle and coronoid process of the ulna	Distal phalanx of fingers 2–5	Finger flexion PIP and DIP and wrist flexion	Median and ulnar
Flexor digitorum superficialis				
Extensor pollicis longus				
Abductor pollicis longus				
Adductor pollicis				

17. Fill in the following chart for measuring range of motion of the hand and wrist. The first one has been done for you as an example.

MOTION	MOVABLE ARM	STATIONARY ARM	FULCRUM	NORMAL RANGE OF MOTION
Wrist flexion	Fifth metacarpal	Ulna	Triquetrum	90 degrees
Wrist extension				
Ulnar deviation				
Radial deviation				

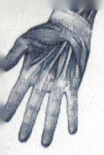

HAND AND WRIST

PALPATION LESSON

You are teaching a lab class on hand and wrist palpation. For the following palpations, explain how you would locate each. The first one has been completed for you.

PALPATION	LOCATION EXPLANATION
1. Lister's tubercle	*Follow the radius in a distal direction to the radial styloid process. Move toward the middle of the hand. Lister's tubercle is about a 1/3 of the way over, even with the third metacarpal.*
2. Triquetrum	
3. TFCC	
4. Extensor pollicis longus	
5. Palmaris longus	
6. Hypothenar eminence	
7. Pisiform	
8. Radial artery	
9. Ulnar collateral ligament of the thumb	

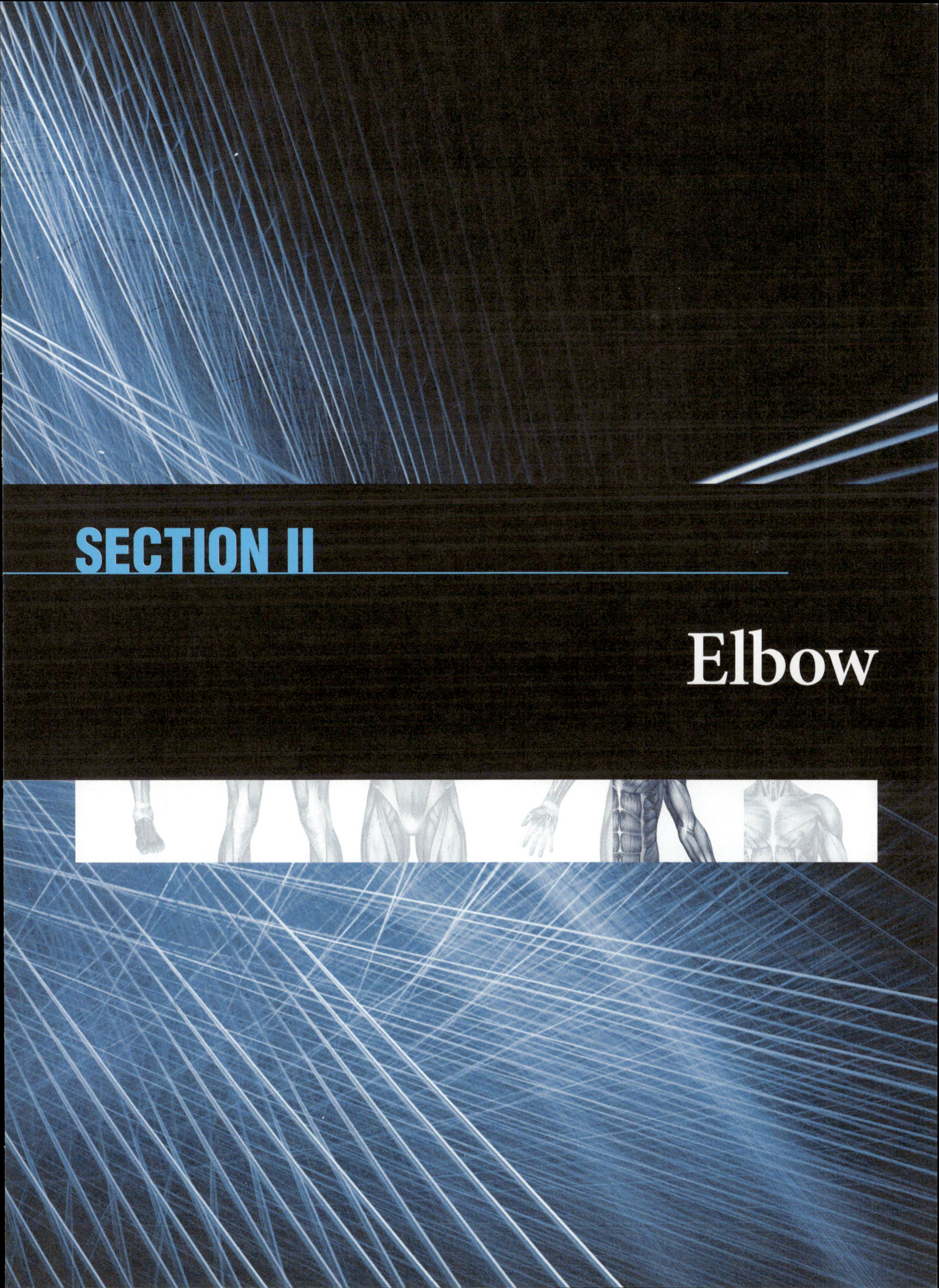

SECTION II

Elbow

LANDMARK IDENTIFICATION

Identify the structures in Figures 2-1 through 2-3. Consult a medical atlas as needed.

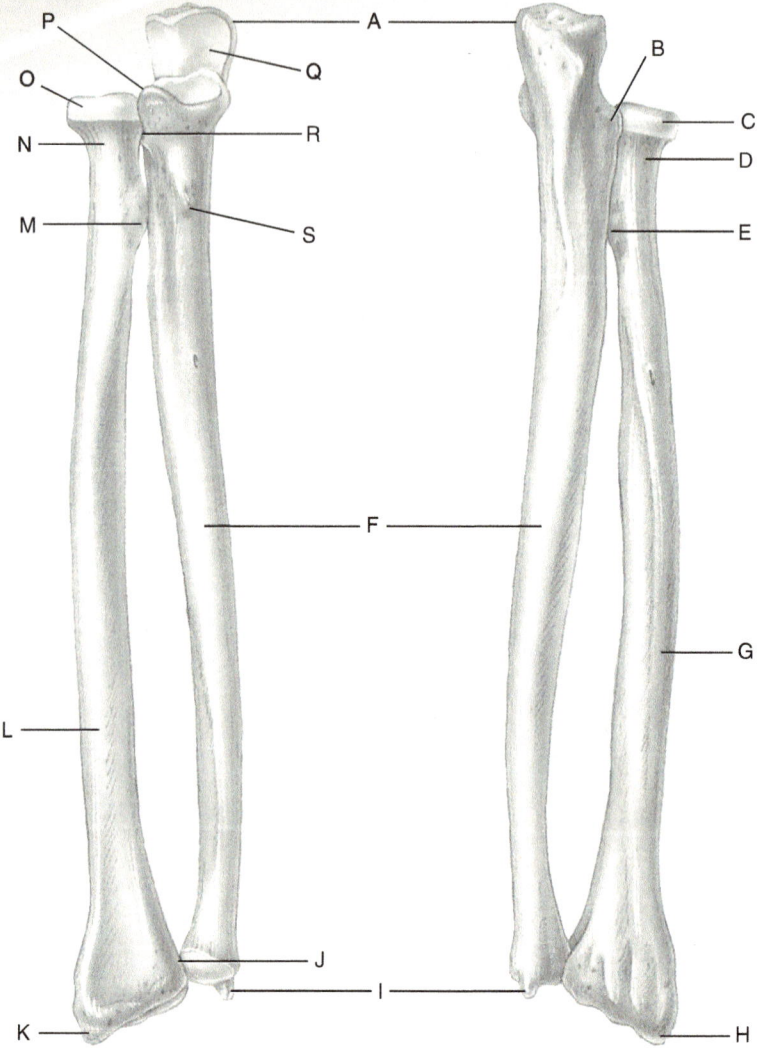

Anterior View   **Posterior View**

FIGURE 2-1

A. _____   K. _____
B. _____   L. _____
C. _____   M. _____
D. _____   N. _____
E. _____   O. _____
F. _____   P. _____
G. _____   Q. _____
H. _____   R. _____
I. _____   S. _____
J. _____

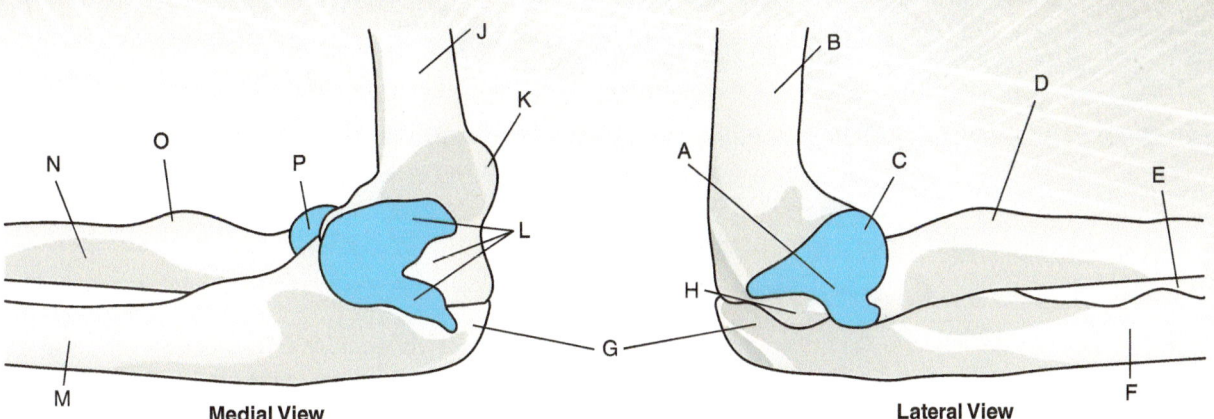

Medial View **Lateral View**

FIGURE 2-2

Lateral View

A. _____ F. _____
B. _____ G. _____
C. _____ H. _____
D. _____ I. _____
E. _____

Medial View

J. _____ N. _____
K. _____ O. _____
L. _____ P. _____
M. _____

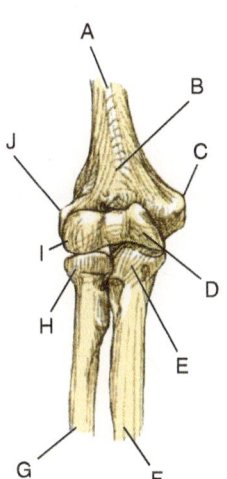

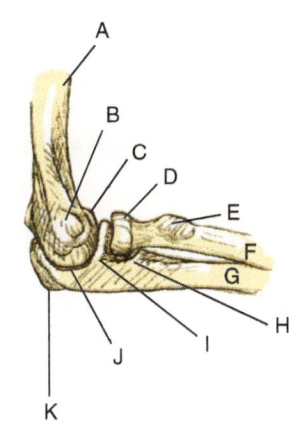

Anterior **Lateral**

FIGURE 2-3

Anterior

A. _____
B. _____
C. _____
D. _____
E. _____
F. _____
G. _____
H. _____
I. _____
J. _____

Lateral

A. _____
B. _____
C. _____
D. _____
E. _____
F. _____
G. _____
H. _____
I. _____
J. _____
K. _____

 # PRACTICAL EXAMINATIONS

Directions: Have another student or professional administer these oral practical examinations. The administrator will read through each list, watch as you perform each task, and mark as you complete it. The person administering the examination should read only the numbered instructions.

PRACTICAL EXAMINATION 1

1. A tennis player is complaining of elbow pain that has gotten progressively worse over the last six weeks. She is now seeking an evaluation from a medical professional. Complete a history for the injury.

QUESTIONS TO ASK PATIENT	COMPLETED (Y/N)/COMMENTS
Where is the pain?	
What kind of pain (for example, numbness, or tingling) are you experiencing?	
What level of pain (from 1 to 10, with 10 being the worst) are you experiencing?	
Are there any movements or activities that make the pain worse, or better?	
What was the mechanism of the injury?	
How did the injury occur?	
When the injury occurred, did you hear any sounds, such as a pop or snap?	
Were you able to keep playing after the injury?	
Have you done or had any treatment for the injury?	
Have you had an injury like this in the past?	
Before the injury, had you recently changed your training or equipment?	
Other pertinent history questions	

2. You are now ready to complete the observation phase of the evaluation. Perform the observation portion of your evaluation, assuming you did not see this individual walk in.

ACTIONS	COMPLETED (Y/N)/COMMENTS
Observe how the patient is holding the injured arm, and the carrying angle	
Check injured area for swelling	
Check injured area for deformity	
Check injured area for discoloration	
Perform bilateral comparison	
Check skin temperature of injured area	
Check muscle tone (anterior, posterior, medial, and lateral)	
Check facial expression for pain	
Other pertinent observations	

3. Palpate the following anatomical landmarks.

PALPATION	COMPLETED (Y/N)/COMMENTS
Medial epicondyle	
Olecranon	
Brachioradialis	
Pronator teres	
Ulnar collateral ligament	
Radial head	

ELBOW

4. Perform the following range of motion tests. (The administrator should mark if each component was done.) Skills should be performed by the examiner unless otherwise noted.

A. Passive Range of Motion for Elbow Flexion

	COMPLETED (Y/N)/COMMENTS
Examiner brings patient's elbow into flexion	
Stabilizes patient's elbow	
Performs test bilaterally	

B. Resistive Range of Motion for Elbow Extension

	COMPLETED (Y/N)/COMMENTS
Provides resistance as patient moves through elbow extension	
Stabilizes patient's elbow	
Performs test bilaterally	

C. Goniometric Test for Forearm Pronation

	COMPLETED (Y/N)/COMMENTS
Has patient's elbow in 90 degrees of flexion	
Has patient in a handshake position	
Places fulcrum on PIP joint of third phalange	
Aligns movement arm pointing straight up towards the ceiling	
Aligns stationary arm perpendicular to the floor	
Measures correctly	

5. Perform the following manual muscle tests. The administrator will check each item as you complete it. Skills should be performed by the examiner unless otherwise noted.

A. Biceps

	COMPLETED (Y/N)/COMMENTS
Stabilizes patient's arm	
Resists elbow flexion	
Performs test bilaterally	
Performs isometric break test	

B. Flexor Carpi Ulnaris

	COMPLETED (Y/N)/COMMENTS
Stabilizes patient's forearm	
Resists elbow flexion toward the ulnar side	
Performs test bilaterally	
Performs isometric break test	

C. Pronator Teres

	COMPLETED (Y/N)/COMMENTS
Stabilizes patient's forearm	
Resists forearm pronation	
Performs test bilaterally	
Performs isometric break test	

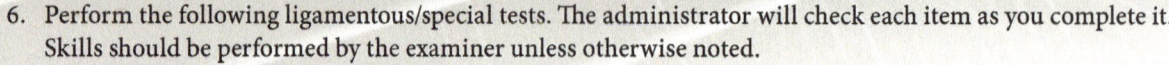

ELBOW

6. Perform the following ligamentous/special tests. The administrator will check each item as you complete it. Skills should be performed by the examiner unless otherwise noted.

A. Valgus Stress Test

	COMPLETED (Y/N)/COMMENTS
Has patient seated	
Stabilizes at patient's elbow	
Patient's elbow flexed 20–30 degrees	
Has one hand at patient's wrist	
Provides adequate valgus force	
Performs test bilaterally	
Understands purpose of valgus stress test and what constitutes a positive test	

B. Tennis Elbow Test

	COMPLETED (Y/N)/COMMENTS
Has patient seated	
Stabilizes at patient's elbow	
Palpates patient's lateral epicondyle	
Has patient extend wrist against resistance	
Understands purpose of tennis elbow test and what constitutes a positive test	

7. Perform a dermatome test for the upper extremity. The administrator will check each item as you complete it.

	COMPLETED (Y/N)/COMMENTS
C1 (top of head)	
C2 (side of face, temple area)	
C3 (angle of mandible)	
C4 (side of neck)	
C5 (proximal humerus, deltoid area)	
C6 (lateral forearm, thumb)	
C7 (middle forearm, 3rd finger)	
C8 (medial forearm, 5th finger)	
T1 (medial humerus)	

PRACTICAL EXAMINATION 2

1. An office worker whose primary job responsibility is re-stocking packages is complaining of elbow pain that has been bothering her on and off for three months. She is now seeking an evaluation from a medical professional. Complete a history for the injury.

QUESTIONS TO ASK PATIENT	COMPLETED (Y/N)/COMMENTS
Where is the pain?	
What kind of pain (for example, numbness, or tingling) are you experiencing?	
What level of pain (from 1 to 10, with 10 being the worst) are you experiencing?	
Are there any movements or activities that make the pain worse, or better?	
What was the mechanism of the injury?	
When you move the elbow, do you hear any sounds, such as a pop or snap?	
Are you able to work and lift boxes?	
Are you experiencing any weakness in the injured area?	
Have you had an injury like this in the past?	
Other pertinent history questions	

ELBOW

2. You are now ready to complete the observation phase of the evaluation. Perform the observation portion of your evaluation, assuming you did not see this individual walk in.

ACTIONS	COMPLETED (Y/N)/COMMENTS
Observe how the patient is holding the injured arm, and the carrying angle	
Check injured area for swelling	
Check injured area for deformity	
Check injured area for discoloration	
Perform bilateral comparison	
Check skin temperature of injured area	
Check muscle tone (anterior, posterior, medial, and lateral)	
Check facial expression for pain	
Other pertinent observations	

3. Palpate the following anatomical landmarks.

PALPATION	COMPLETED (Y/N)/COMMENTS
Ulnar nerve	
Triceps	
Palmaris longus	
Lateral collateral ligament	
Flexor carpi radialis	
Radial styloid process	

4. Perform the following range of motion tests. (The administrator should mark if each component was done.) Skills should be performed by the examiner unless otherwise noted.

A. Active Range of Motion for Forearm Supination

	COMPLETED (Y/N)/COMMENTS
Has client move forearm into supination	
Stabilizes patient's arm	
Performs test bilaterally	

B. Goniometric Test for Elbow Flexion

	COMPLETED (Y/N)/COMMENTS
Places fulcrum with lateral epicondyle	
Aligns stationary arm with lateral humerus	
Aligns movement arm with radius	
Measures correctly	

5. Perform the following manual muscle tests. The administrator will check each item as you complete it. Skills should be performed by the examiner unless otherwise noted.

A. Brachioradialis

	COMPLETED (Y/N)/COMMENTS
Stabilizes patient's arm	
Resists elbow flexion with forearm in neutral position	
Performs test bilaterally	
Performs isometric break test	

B. Extensor Carpi Radialis Longus

	COMPLETED (Y/N)/COMMENTS
Stabilizes patient's forearm	
Resists elbow extension toward the radial side	
Performs test bilaterally	
Performs isometric break test	

C. Triceps

	COMPLETED (Y/N)/COMMENTS
Stabilizes patient's arm	
Resists elbow extension	
Performs test bilaterally	
Performs isometric break test	

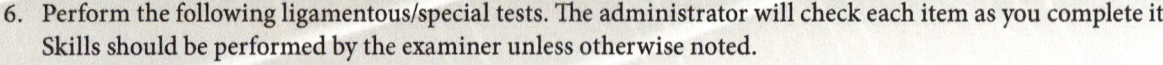
ELBOW

6. Perform the following ligamentous/special tests. The administrator will check each item as you complete it. Skills should be performed by the examiner unless otherwise noted.

   A. Varus Stress Test

	COMPLETED (Y/N)/COMMENTS
Stabilizes arm at elbow	
Has patient seated	
Patient's elbow flexed 20–30 degrees	
Has one hand at patient's wrist	
Provides adequate varus force	
Performs test bilaterally	
Understands purpose of varus stress test and what constitutes a positive test	

   B. Tinel's Sign (Ulnar Nerve)

	COMPLETED (Y/N)/COMMENTS
Stabilizes the patient's forearm	
Taps on the patient's ulnar nerve in ulnar notch	
Understands purpose of Tinel's sign and what constitutes a positive test	

7. Perform a myotome test for the upper extremity. The administrator will check each item as you complete it.

	COMPLETED (Y/N)/COMMENTS
C1 (neck flexion)	
C2 (neck flexion)	
C3 (neck lateral flexion)	
C4 (shoulder elevation)	
C5 (shoulder abduction)	
C6 (elbow flexion, wrist extension)	
C7 (elbow extension, wrist flexion)	
C8 (thumb extension)	
T1 (finger abduction, adduction)	

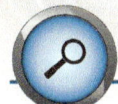 ## SCAVENGER HUNT

Read the following questions and try to find the answers by watching the CD enclosed with this text.

1. How can you make the radial head more prominent?

_____

_____

2. When placing the palm of the hand on the medial epicondyle, what does the index finger point to?

_____

_____

3. What is the normal range of motion for forearm pronation?

_____

_____

4. The forearm is placed in what position when testing the brachioradialis?

_____

_____

5. How many degrees is the elbow flexed when a valgus or varus stress test is performed?

_____

_____

6. Tinel's sign for the elbow is done for which nerve?

_____

_____

7. Describe where the nerve from Question 6 is located.

_____

_____

8. How many muscles mentioned in the elbow section are responsible for elbow extension?

_____

_____

9. What mechanisms of injury are mentioned for an MCL sprain?

_____

_____

10. What structure is palpated during the tennis elbow test?

_____

_____

 # PEER ASSESSMENTS

Ask a fellow classmate or peer to assess your performance of the following evaluation procedures. After the assessment is completed, answer the post-assessment questions on your own. When you feel confident in your proficiency, you may want to re-test your performance of these skills with a professional acting as your peer reviewer.

PEER ASSESSMENT 1

EVALUATION SKILLS	DATE OF ASSESSMENT	CORRECT/NOT CORRECT	COMMENTS
Palpations Olecranon Lateral epicondyle Ulnar nerve Palmaris longus			
Range of Motion Active flexion Passive supination Goniometric measurement pronation			
Manual Muscle Tests Flexor carpi radialis Biceps Extensor carpi ulnaris			
Ligamentous/Special Tests Valgus stress test Tinel's sign			
Neurological Tests Dermatome assessment upper extremity C1–T1			

Reviewer's Signature: _____ Date: _____

Post-Assessment Questions

1. Did you feel confident during the peer assessment?

   _____

2. Which skills (manual muscle tests, range of motion, etc.) did you feel most confident completing, and why?

   _____

3. Which skill did you feel least confident completing, and why?

   _____

PEER ASSESSMENT 2

Perform this assessment at least two weeks after completing Peer Assessment 1. Follow the directions provided for the first peer assessment.

EVALUATION SKILLS	DATE OF ASSESSMENT	CORRECT/NOT CORRECT	COMMENTS
Palpations Radial head Medial collateral ligament Ulna Pronator teres			
Range of Motion Active pronation Passive flexion Goniometric measurement extension			
Manual Muscle Tests Brachioradialis Triceps Supinator			
Ligamentous/Special Tests Varus stress test Tennis elbow test			
Neurological Tests Myotome assessment upper extremity C1–T1			
Reviewer's Signature: _____ Date: _____			

ELBOW

Post-Assessment Questions

1. Do you feel more comfortable with the evaluation of the elbow than you did during the first assessment? Why or why not?

_____

_____

2. In which area (manual muscle tests, special tests, etc.) do you have the most confidence in your abilities, and why?

_____

_____

3. In which area do you feel the least confident in your abilities, and why?

_____

_____

4. Name three palpations of the elbow that you have no difficulty locating. (Note: these do not need to be palpations discussed in this assessment.)

_____

_____

5. Name three palpations of the elbow that tend to be challenging for you to find. (Note: these do not need to be palpations discussed in this assessment.)

_____

_____

PEER ASSESSMENT 3

Perform this assessment at least two weeks after completing Peer Assessment 2. This assessment should take longer than Assessments 1 and 2. Ask a fellow classmate or peer to develop their own questions in the following categories and assess your performance. After the peer assessment is completed, answer the post-assessment questions on your own. When you feel confident with your proficiency, you may want to re-test your performance of these skills with a professional acting as your peer reviewer.

EVALUATION SKILLS	DATE OF ASSESSMENT	CORRECT/ NOT CORRECT	COMMENTS
Palpations of the elbow			
Range of motion of the elbow			
Manual muscle tests of the elbow			
Ligamentous/special tests of the elbow			
Neurological tests of the elbow			
Reviewer's Signature: _____ Date: _____			

Post-Assessment Questions

1. Do you feel competent in performing an evaluation of the elbow in order to reach a diagnosis?

   _____

   _____

2. With regards to the elbow, what do you feel is the most important part of the injury evaluation process, and why?

   _____

   _____

3. How have your evaluation skills improved from the first assessment to the third?

   _____

   _____

4. How can you continue to improve your evaluation skills?

   _____

   _____

SPECIAL TEST SUB-SKILLS

For the special tests listed, write out the sub-skills necessary for skill completion. In addition, list what pathology each special test is checking for and what constitutes a positive test. The first one has been done for you as an example.

TEST	SUB-SKILLS	STRUCTURE(S) TESTED	POSITIVE TEST INDICATIONS
Valgus stress	• Has client's elbow flexed to 20–30 degrees • Stabilizes at elbow laterally • Has hand at wrist medially • Has client relax • Applies valgus force • Performs test bilaterally	This test is for the medial collateral ligament of the elbow.	A positive test is indicated by pain and/or laxity in the elbow.
Varus stress			
Tinel's sign			
Tennis elbow test			

Complete the below exercise for four additional special/ligament tests.

TEST	SUB-SKILLS	STRUCTURE(S) TESTED	POSITIVE TEST INDICATION

RELATED ELBOW QUESTIONS

1. The normal carrying angle of the elbow in women is between _____ and _____ degrees.

2. The wrist extensor group of muscles originates on the _____.

3. The primary resistance to a valgus force placed on the elbow is the _____.

4. The _____ is the most frequently injured bursa in the elbow.

5. Pitcher's elbow and little league elbow affect the _____ (an anatomical structure).

6. A 3 out of 5 grade on a triceps manual muscle test means that the elbow _____
   _____.

7. When a client is diagnosed with a grade II MCL sprain of the elbow, his signs and symptoms likely include _____
   _____.

8. The elbow joint is made of _____ bones.

9. Fill in the following chart for each muscle of the elbow. The first one has been done for you.

MUSCLE	ORIGIN	INSERTION	ACTION	INNERVATION
Biceps brachii (long head)	Supraglenoid tubercle of scapula	Radial tuberosity of radius	Flexion elbow and arm and supination of forearm	Musculocutaneous
Triceps brachii (long head)				
Brachialis				
Pronator teres				
Flexor carpi radialis				

10. Fill in the following chart for measuring range of motion of the elbow. The first one has been done for you as an example.

MOTION	MOVABLE ARM	STATIONARY ARM	FULCRUM	NORMAL RANGE OF MOTION
Elbow flexion	Radius	Lateral humerus	Lateral epicondyle	140–150 degrees
Elbow extension				
Pronation				
Supination				

ELBOW

PALPATION LESSON

You are teaching a lab class on elbow palpation. For the following palpations, explain how you would locate each. The first one has been completed for you.

PALPATION	LOCATION EXPLANATION
1. Olecranon	*This is the rounded part of the elbow located on the posterior surface. Start at the anterior cubital fossa and palpate the rounded posterior surface (which is the olecranon).*
2. Ulnar nerve	
3. Pronator teres	
4. Radial head	
5. Brachioradialis	
6. Lateral epicondyle	
7. Medial collateral ligament	
8. Brachial artery	

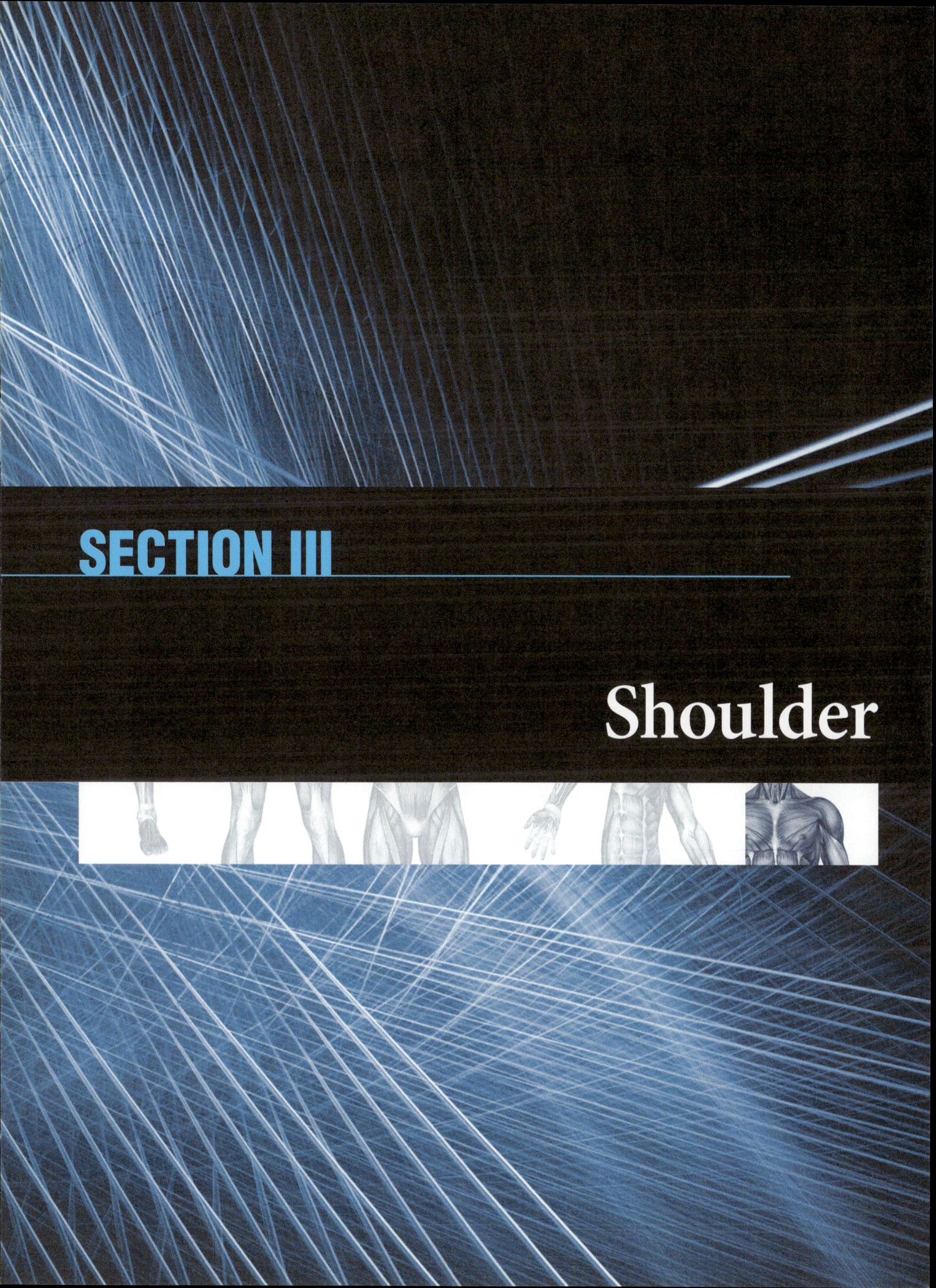

SECTION III

Shoulder

LANDMARK IDENTIFICATION

Identify the structures in Figures 3-1 through 3-5. Consult a medical atlas as needed.

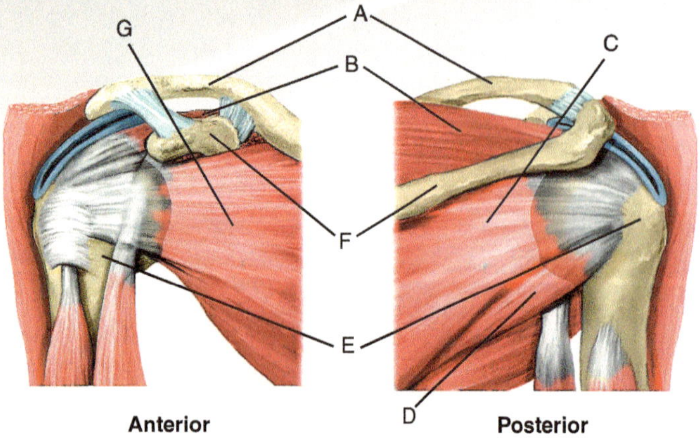

Anterior

Posterior

FIGURE 3-1

A. _____   E. _____

B. _____   F. _____

C. _____   G. _____

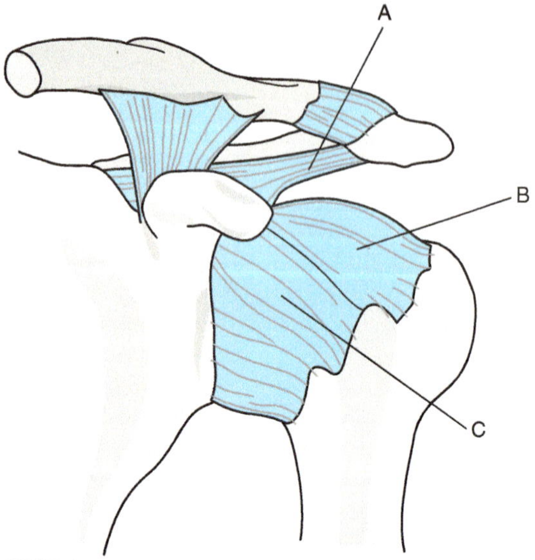

D. _____

FIGURE 3-2

A. _____

B. _____

C. _____

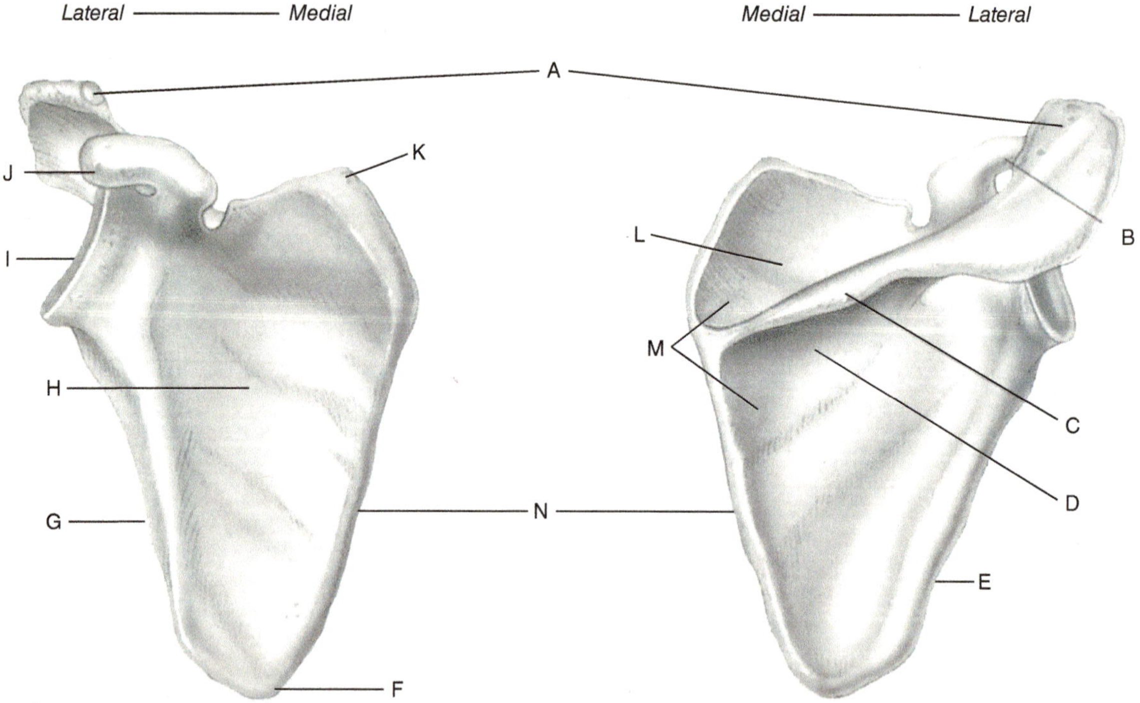

Lateral ——————— *Medial*   *Medial* ——————— *Lateral*

FIGURE 3-3

A. _____   D. _____   G. _____   J. _____   M. _____

B. _____   E. _____   H. _____   K. _____   N. _____

C. _____   F. _____   I. _____   L. _____

SHOULDER

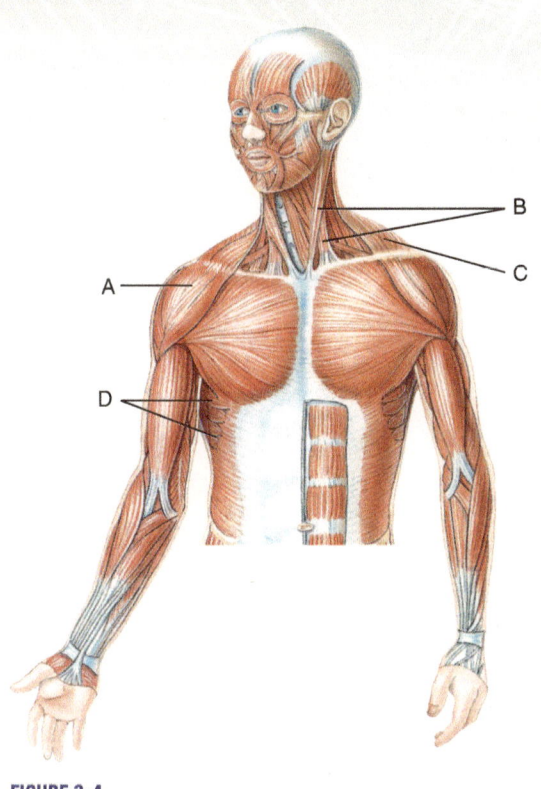

FIGURE 3-4

A. _____
B. _____
C. _____
D. _____

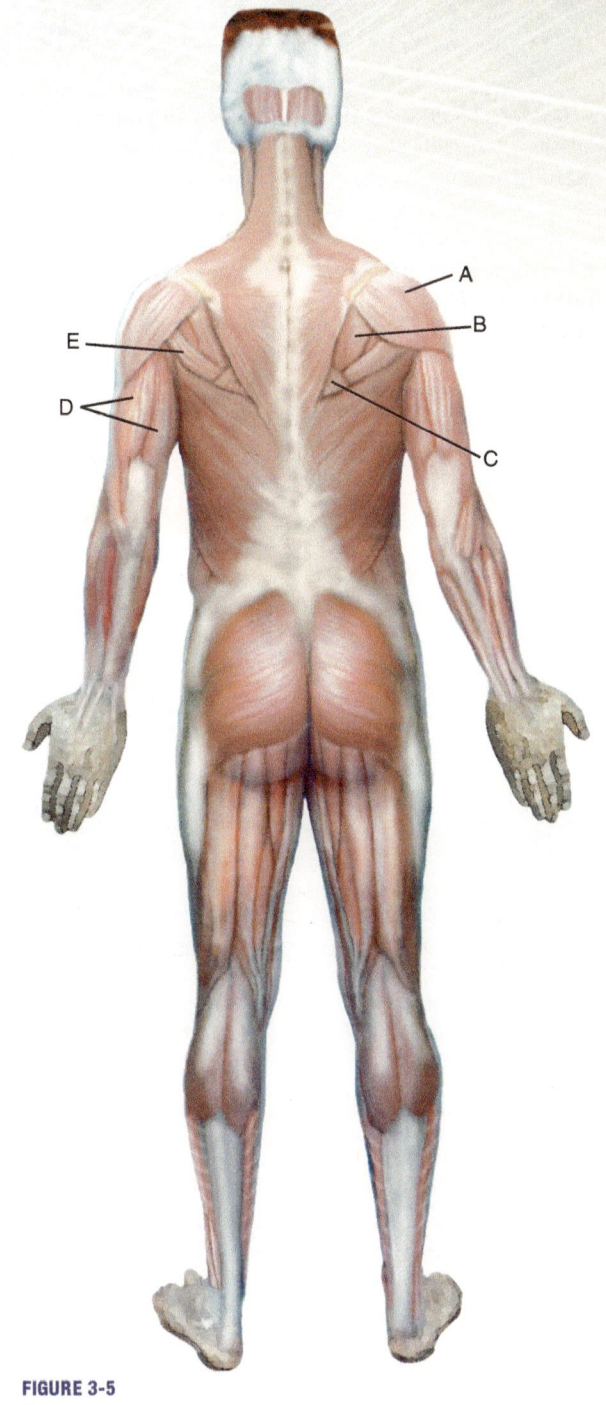

FIGURE 3-5

A. _____
B. _____
C. _____
D. _____
E. _____

 # PRACTICAL EXAMINATIONS

Directions: Have another student or professional administer these oral practical examinations. The administrator of the exam will read through each list, watch as you perform each task, and mark as you complete it. The person administering the examination should read only the numbered instructions.

PRACTICAL EXAMINATION 1

1. A swimmer hurt his shoulder in a meet two weeks ago. The injury has gotten progressively worse, and he is now in your athletic training room, seeking an evaluation. Complete a history for the injury.

QUESTIONS TO ASK PATIENT	COMPLETED (Y/N)/COMMENTS
Where is the pain?	
What kind of pain (for example, numbness, or tingling) are you experiencing?	
What level of pain (from 1 to 10, with 10 being the worst) are you experiencing?	
Are there any movements or activities that make the pain worse, or better?	
When the injury occurred, did you hear any sounds, such as a pop or snap? Do you hear any sounds when you move your shoulder now?	
What was the mechanism of injury?	
Were you able to keep playing on the injury?	
Have you done or had any treatment for the injury?	
Have you had an injury like this in the past?	
Before the injury, had you recently changed your training or equipment?	
Other pertinent history questions	

2. You are now ready to complete the observation phase of the evaluation. Perform the observation portion of your evaluation, assuming you did not see this individual walk in.

ACTIONS	COMPLETED (Y/N)/COMMENTS
Observe how the patient is holding the injured arm, and the carrying angle	
Check injured area for swelling	
Check injured area for deformity	
Check injured area for discoloration	
Perform bilateral comparison	
Check muscle tone (anterior, posterior, medial, and lateral)	
Check scapular position and level of shoulders	
Check skin temperature of injured area	
Check facial expression for pain	
Other pertinent observations	

3. Palpate the following anatomical landmarks.

PALPATION	COMPLETED (Y/N)/COMMENTS
Sternoclavicular (SC) joint	
Clavicle	
Àcromioclavicular (AC) joint	
Spine of the scapula	
Greater tuberosity	
Deltoid tuberosity	
Infraspinous fossa	
Coracoid process	

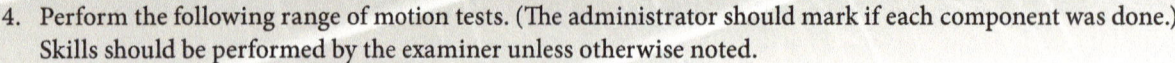

SHOULDER

4. Perform the following range of motion tests. (The administrator should mark if each component was done.) Skills should be performed by the examiner unless otherwise noted.

A. Passive Range of Motion for Shoulder Flexion

	COMPLETED (Y/N)/COMMENTS
Brings patient's shoulder into flexion	
Stabilizes patient's shoulder	
Performs test bilaterally	

B. Resistive Range of Motion for Shoulder Abduction

	COMPLETED (Y/N)/COMMENTS
Provides resistance as patient moves through shoulder abduction	
Stabilizes patient's shoulder	
Performs test bilaterally	

C. Goniometric Test for Shoulder External Rotation

	COMPLETED (Y/N)/COMMENTS
Places fulcrum on olecranon	
Aligns stationary arm perpendicular to floor	
Aligns movement arm with forearm	
Measures correctly	

5. Perform the following manual muscle tests. The administrator will check each item as you complete it. Skills should be performed by the examiner unless otherwise noted.

A. Middle Trapezius

	COMPLETED (Y/N)/COMMENTS
Stabilizes patient's shoulder	
Resists horizontal abduction with external rotation	
Performs test bilaterally	
Performs isometric break test	

B. Supraspinatus

	COMPLETED (Y/N)/COMMENTS
Stabilizes patient's shoulder	
Resists abduction	
Performs test bilaterally	
Performs isometric break test	

C. Infraspinatus

	COMPLETED (Y/N)/COMMENTS
Stabilizes patient's shoulder	
Resists external rotation	
Performs test bilaterally	
Performs isometric break test	

D. Pectoralis Minor

	COMPLETED (Y/N)/COMMENTS
Stabilizes patient's shoulder	
Resists protraction	
Performs test bilaterally	
Performs isometric break test	

E. Rhomboids

	COMPLETED (Y/N)/COMMENTS
Stabilizes patient's shoulder	
Resists retraction	
Performs test bilaterally	
Performs isometric break test	

6. Perform the following ligamentous/special tests. The administrator will check each item as you complete it. Skills should be performed by the examiner unless otherwise noted.

A. Apprehension Test

	COMPLETED (Y/N)/COMMENTS
Stabilizes patient's shoulder	
Has patient in supine position, with shoulder slightly off table	
Has patient relax	
Moves patient into 90-degree abduction and external rotation	
Performs test bilaterally	
Has hands in appropriate position	
Understands purpose of apprehension test and what constitutes a positive test	

B. Empty Can Test

	COMPLETED (Y/N)/COMMENTS
Has patient sitting or standing with shoulders adducted to 90 degrees, horizontally adducted to 30 degrees with full internal rotation	
Places resistance on patient's distal arm	
Resists shoulder abduction	
Understands purpose of empty can test and what constitutes a positive test	

C. Sternoclavicular Joint Stress Test

	COMPLETED (Y/N)/COMMENTS
Has patient in seated position	
Places hand on patient's proximal clavicle and spine of scapula	
Has patient relax shoulder	
Applies **downward** and inward force on the clavicle	
Performs test bilaterally	
Understands purpose of sternoclavicular joint stress test and what constitutes a positive test	

D. Speed's Test

	COMPLETED (Y/N)/COMMENTS
Has patient seated or standing, with shoulder flexed to 90 degrees and forearm in supination	
Places one hand on patient's proximal humerus near bicipital groove	
Places other hand on patient's distal forearm	
Resists shoulder flexion	
Performs test bilaterally	
Understands purpose of Speed's test and what constitutes a positive test	

E. Feagin's Test

	COMPLETED (Y/N)/COMMENTS
Has patient in seated position	
Abducts patient's shoulder to 90 degrees and rests it on top of examiner's shoulder	
Interlocks hands and places them over patient's proximal humerus	
Applies downward force on patient's proximal humerus	
Performs test bilaterally	
Understands purpose of Feagin's test and what constitutes a positive test	

7. Perform a dermatome test for the upper extremity. The administrator will check each item as you complete it.

	COMPLETED (Y/N)/COMMENTS
C1 (top of head)	
C2 (side of face, temple area)	
C3 (angle of mandible)	
C4 (side of neck)	
C5 (proximal humerus, deltoid area)	
C6 (lateral forearm, thumb)	
C7 (middle forearm, 3rd finger)	
C8 (medial forearm, 5th finger)	
T1 (medial humerus)	

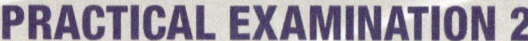
SHOULDER

PRACTICAL EXAMINATION 2

1. A softball player comes into your athletic training room complaining of shoulder pain that first occurred yesterday at practice. They are now seeking an evaluation from a medical professional. Complete a history for the injury.

QUESTIONS TO ASK PATIENT	COMPLETED (Y/N)/COMMENTS
Where is the pain?	
What kind of pain (for example, numbness, or tingling) are you experiencing?	
What level of pain (from 1 to 10, with 10 being the worst) are you experiencing?	
Are there any movements or activities that make the pain worse, or better?	
What was the mechanism of injury?	
When you move the shoulder, do you hear any sounds, such as a pop or snap? Did you hear any sounds when it was first injured?	
Were you able to keep playing after the injury?	
Have you done or had any treatment for the injury?	
Have you had an injury like this in the past?	
Before the injury, had you recently changed your training or equipment?	
Other pertinent history questions	

2. You are now ready to complete the observation phase of the evaluation. Perform the observation portion of your evaluation, assuming you did not see this individual walk in.

ACTIONS	COMPLETED (Y/N)/COMMENTS
Observe how the patient is holding the injured arm, and the carrying angle	
Check injured area for swelling	
Check injured area for deformity	
Check injured area for discoloration	
Perform bilateral comparison	
Check muscle tone (anterior, posterior, medial, and lateral)	
Check skin temperature of injured area	
Check facial expression for pain	
Check scapular position and level of shoulders	
Other pertinent observations	

3. Palpate the following anatomical landmarks.

PALPATION	COMPLETED (Y/N)/COMMENTS
Coracoid process	
Bicipital groove	
Latissimus dorsi	
Subacromial bursa	
Pectoralis major	
Rhomboids	

SHOULDER

4. Perform the following range of motion tests. (The administrator should mark if each component was done.) Skills should be performed by the examiner unless otherwise noted.

   A. Resistive Range of Motion for Shoulder External Rotation

	COMPLETED (Y/N)/COMMENTS
Provides resistance as patient moves through shoulder external rotation	
Stabilizes patient's shoulder	
Performs test bilaterally	

   B. Goniometric Measurement for Shoulder Extension

	COMPLETED (Y/N)/COMMENTS
Has patient properly positioned	
Places fulcrum on acromion	
Aligns stationary arm with torso midline	
Aligns movement arm with the humerus	
Performs test bilaterally	
Measures correctly	

5. Perform the following manual muscle test for the following muscles. The administrator will check each item as you complete it. Skills should be performed by the examiner unless otherwise noted.

   A. Pectoralis Minor

	COMPLETED (Y/N)/COMMENTS
Has patient in supine position	
Instructs patient to protract shoulder	
Stabilizes patient's torso	
Resists shoulder protraction	
Performs test bilaterally	
Performs isometric break test	

B. Coracobrachialis

	COMPLETED (Y/N)/COMMENTS
Has patient seated, with elbow in full flexion	
Instructs patient to place shoulder in slight flexion	
Stabilizes patient's shoulder	
Resists shoulder flexion	
Performs test bilaterally	
Performs isometric break test	

C. Teres Major

	COMPLETED (Y/N)/COMMENTS
Patient prone with dorsal surface of hand placed on posterior iliac crest	
Instructs patient to maintain test position	
Stabilizes patient's shoulder	
Resists extension and adduction	
Performs test bilaterally	
Performs isometric break test	

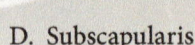

SHOULDER

D. Subscapularis

	COMPLETED (Y/N)/COMMENTS
Has patient seated or standing, with elbow flexed to 90 degrees	
Instructs patient to internally rotate shoulder	
Stabilizes patient's distal humerus	
Resists shoulder internal rotation	
Performs test bilaterally	
Performs isometric break test	

E. Serratus Anterior

	COMPLETED (Y/N)/COMMENTS
Has patient in supine position, with shoulder flexed to 90 degrees	
Instructs patient to protract shoulder	
Stabilizes patient's torso	
Resists shoulder protraction	
Performs test bilaterally	
Performs isometric break test	

6. Perform the following ligamentous/special tests. The administrator will check each item as you complete it. Skills should be performed by the examiner unless otherwise noted.

A. Neer Impingement Test

	COMPLETED (Y/N)/COMMENTS
Has patient in seated position	
Uses one hand to stabilize patient's scapula	
Uses other hand to hold patient's distal humerus	
Has patient relax shoulder	
Passively moves patient's involved shoulder into full flexion	
Performs test bilaterally	
Understands purpose of Neer impingement test and what constitutes a positive test	

B. Yergason's Test

	COMPLETED (Y/N)/COMMENTS
Has patient in seated position, with elbow flexed to 90 degrees and forearm in full pronation	
Uses one hand to stabilize patient's humerus	
Places other hand on patient's distal forearm	
Resists supination and external rotation	
Performs test bilaterally	
Understands purpose of Yergason's test and what constitutes a positive test	

C. Posterior Drawer Test

	COMPLETED (Y/N)/COMMENTS
Has patient in supine position	
Uses one hand to stabilize patient's scapula, with fingers on spine of scapula and thumb on coracoid process	
Uses other hand to hold patient's distal humerus	
Has patient relax shoulder	
Passively abducts patient's shoulder to 90 degrees, horizontally adducts patient's shoulder to 20–30 degrees	
Internally rotates patient's shoulder	
Applies downward pressure, gliding the patient's humeral head in posterior direction	
Performs test bilaterally	
Understands purpose of posterior drawer test and what constitutes a positive test	

SHOULDER

D. O'Brien's Test

	COMPLETED (Y/N)/COMMENTS
Has patient in seated position or standing	
Has patient's shoulder flexed to 90 degrees, horizontally adducted to 30–45 degrees, with maximal internal rotation	
Uses one hand to stabilize patient's shoulder	
Places other hand on patient's wrist	
Applies downward force on patient's arm	
Notes any pain or clicking	
Moves patient's shoulder into full external rotation	
Reapplies downward force on patient's arm	
Performs test bilaterally	
Understands purpose of O'Brien's Test and what constitutes a positive test	

E. Brachial Plexus Stretch Test

	COMPLETED (Y/N)/COMMENTS
Has patient in seated position or standing	
Stands behind patient	
Places one hand on patient's shoulder	
Places other hand on side of subject's head	
Laterally flexes patient's head away	
Applies downward force on patient's shoulder	
Performs test bilaterally	
Understands purpose of brachial plexus stretch test and what constitutes a positive test	

7. Perform a myotome test for the upper extremity. The administrator will check each item as you complete it.

	COMPLETED (Y/N)/COMMENTS
C1 (neck flexion)	
C2 (neck flexion)	
C3 (neck lateral flexion)	
C4 (shoulder elevation)	
C5 (shoulder abduction)	
C6 (elbow flexion, wrist extension)	
C7 (elbow extension, wrist flexion)	
C8 (thumb extension, ulnar deviation)	
T1 (finger abduction, adduction)	

 # SCAVENGER HUNT

Read the following questions and try to find the answers by watching the CD enclosed with this text.

1. How can you make the lesser tuberosity more prominent?

_____

_____

2. What does the term SLAP lesion refer to?

_____

_____

SHOULDER

3. What muscles are involved with impingement syndrome?

_____

_____

4. A patient sustains an AC joint sprain. What specific areas would be important to palpate? What special/ ligamentous tests could be done to help determine ligament stability?

_____

_____

5. What is a stinger?

_____

_____

6. If someone is suffering from biceps tendonitis, where would she be experiencing pain?

_____

_____

7. Where do the majority of clavicle fractures occur?

_____

_____

8. What is the normal range of motion in degrees for shoulder flexion?

_____

_____

9. What does the term GIRD stand for?

_____

_____

10. Name all the special tests that could be used to diagnose glenohumeral joint instability.

_____

_____

 # PEER ASSESSMENTS

Ask a fellow classmate or peer to assess your performance of the following evaluation procedures. After the assessment is completed, answer the post-assessment questions on your own. When you feel confident in your proficiency, you may want to re-test your performance of these skills with a professional acting as your peer reviewer.

PEER ASSESSMENT 1

EVALUATION SKILLS	DATE OF ASSESSMENT	CORRECT/NOT CORRECT	COMMENTS
Palpations SC joint Acromion Spine of scapula Coracoid process Sternocleidomastoid			

Range of Motion
Goniometric measurement
  for internal rotation
Resistive range of motion
  for horizontal adduction			

Manual Muscle Tests Pectoralis major Serratus anterior Lower trapezius			
Ligamentous/Special Tests Anterior drawer test Yergason test Speed's test			
Neurological Tests Dermatome assessment upper extremity C1–T1 C5 reflex			

Reviewer's Signature: _____ Date: _____

Post-Assessment Questions

1. Did you feel confident during the peer assessment?

_____

2. Which skills (manual muscle tests, range of motion, etc.) did you feel most confident completing, and why?

_____

3. Which skill did you feel least confident completing, and why?

_____

PEER ASSESSMENT 2

Perform this assessment at least two weeks after completing Peer Assessment 1. Follow the directions provided for the first peer assessment.

EVALUATION SKILLS	DATE OF ASSESSMENT	CORRECT/NOT CORRECT	COMMENTS
Palpations Superior angle of scapula Deltoid tuberosity Bicipital groove AC joint			
Range of Motion Goniometric measurement for shoulder flexion Passive range of motion shoulder extension			
Manual Muscle Tests Deltoid Teres major Upper trapezius			
Ligamentous/Special Tests Empty can test Posterior apprehension test O'Brien's test			
Neurological Tests Myotome assessment upper extremity C1–T1			
Reviewer's Signature: _____		Date: _____	

Post-Assessment Questions

1. Do you feel more comfortable with the evaluation of the shoulder than you did during the first assessment? Why or why not?

   _____

   _____

2. In which area (manual muscle tests, special tests, etc.) do you have the most confidence in your abilities, and why?

   _____

   _____

3. In which area do you feel the least confident in your abilities, and why?

   _____

   _____

4. Name three palpations of the shoulder that you have no difficulty locating. (Note: these do not need to be palpations discussed in this assessment.)

   _____

   _____

5. Name three palpations of the shoulder that tend to be challenging for you to find. (Note: these do not need to be palpations discussed in this assessment.)

   _____

   _____

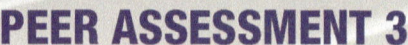

SHOULDER

PEER ASSESSMENT 3

Perform this assessment at least two weeks after completing Peer Assessment 2. This assessment should take longer than Assessments 1 and 2. Ask a fellow classmate or peer to develop their own questions in the following categories and assess your performance. After the peer assessment is completed, answer the post-assessment questions on your own. When you feel confident with your proficiency, you may want to re-test your performance of these skills with a professional acting as your peer reviewer.

EVALUATION SKILLS	DATE OF ASSESSMENT	CORRECT/ NOT CORRECT	COMMENTS
Palpations of the shoulder			
Range of motion of the shoulder			
Manual muscle tests for the shoulder			
Ligamentous/special tests for the shoulder			
Neurological tests for the shoulder			

Reviewer's Signature: _____ Date: _____

Post-Assessment Questions

1. Do you feel competent in performing an evaluation of the shoulder to find a diagnosis?

   _____

   _____

2. With regards to the shoulder, what do you feel is the most important part of the injury evaluation process, and why?

   _____

   _____

3. How have your evaluation skills improved from the first assessment to the third?

   _____

   _____

4. How can you to continue to improve your evaluation skills?

   _____

   _____

SPECIAL TEST SUB-SKILLS

For the special tests listed, write out the sub-skills necessary for skill completion. In addition, list what each special test is for and what constitutes a positive test. The first one has been done for you as an example.

TEST	SUB-SKILLS	STRUCTURE(S) TESTED	POSITIVE TEST INDICATIONS
Posterior drawer	• *Has patient supine* • *Abducts patient's shoulder 90 degrees* • *Places patient's shoulder in 20–30 degrees horizontal flexion* • *Stabilizes patient's scapula and places thumb over coracoid process* • *Places Posterior force on humerus*	*This test is used to check for instability of the glenohumeral joint (posterior).*	*A positive test is indicated by pain and/or laxity in the shoulder.*
Cross-over impingement			
Neer impingement			
Drop arm			

Complete the below exercise for four additional special/ligament tests.

TEST	SUB-SKILLS	STRUCTURE(S) TESTED	POSITIVE TEST INDICATIONS

SHOULDER

RELATED SHOULDER QUESTIONS

1. The shoulder girdle is made up of which three joints? _____

2. The _____ can be a common site for Myositis ossificans in the shoulder.

3. The spine of the scapula is at the same level as the _____ spinous process.

4. The inferior angle of the scapula is at the same level as the _____.

5. If you suspect a patient is suffering from impingement syndrome, you would likely perform the _____, _____, and _____ tests.

6. To differentiate the injured structure when performing an AC joint distraction test, you should note if _____.

7. The piano key sign will be positive if a patient is suffering from _____, in the _____ grade of the injury.

8. When performing the _____ test, you observe the patient is unable to slowly lower his or her arm from full abduction, indicating he or she is suffering from a _____.

9. After completing an evaluation, you grade the strength of a patient's deltoid as a 4, meaning the deltoid _____.

10. Erb's point is located _____, the area where the _____.

11. Fill in the following chart for each muscle of the shoulder. The first one has been done for you.

MUSCLE	ORIGIN	INSERTION	ACTION	INNERVATION
Deltoid (anterior)	Lateral 1/3 of clavicle, anterior superior surface	Deltoid tuberosity of humerus	Abduction, flexion and medial rotation	Axillary
Pectoralis major (sternal)				
Teres minor				
Levator scapulae				
Latissimus dorsi				
Rhomboid minor				
Supraspinatus				

12. Fill in the following chart for measuring range of motion of the shoulder. The first one has been done for you as an example.

MOTION	MOVZABLE ARM	STATIONARY ARM	FULCRUM	NORMAL RANGE OF MOTION
Shoulder extension	Lateral humerus	Lateral torso parallel to mid-line	Acromium	50–60 degrees
Shoulder flexion				
Shoulder internal rotation				
Shoulder external rotation				

PALPATION LESSON

You are teaching a lab class on shoulder palpation. For the following palpations, explain how you would locate each. The first one has been completed for you.

PALPATION	LOCATION EXPLANATION
1. AC joint	Follow the clavicle out to the acromioclavicular joint, also known as the AC joint. This is where the acromion and the clavicle articulate.
2. Spine of scapula	
3. Bicipital groove	
4. Deltoid tuberosity	
5. Subacromial bursa	
6. Lateral border of the scapula	
7. Sternal notch	
8. Lesser tuberosity of humerus	

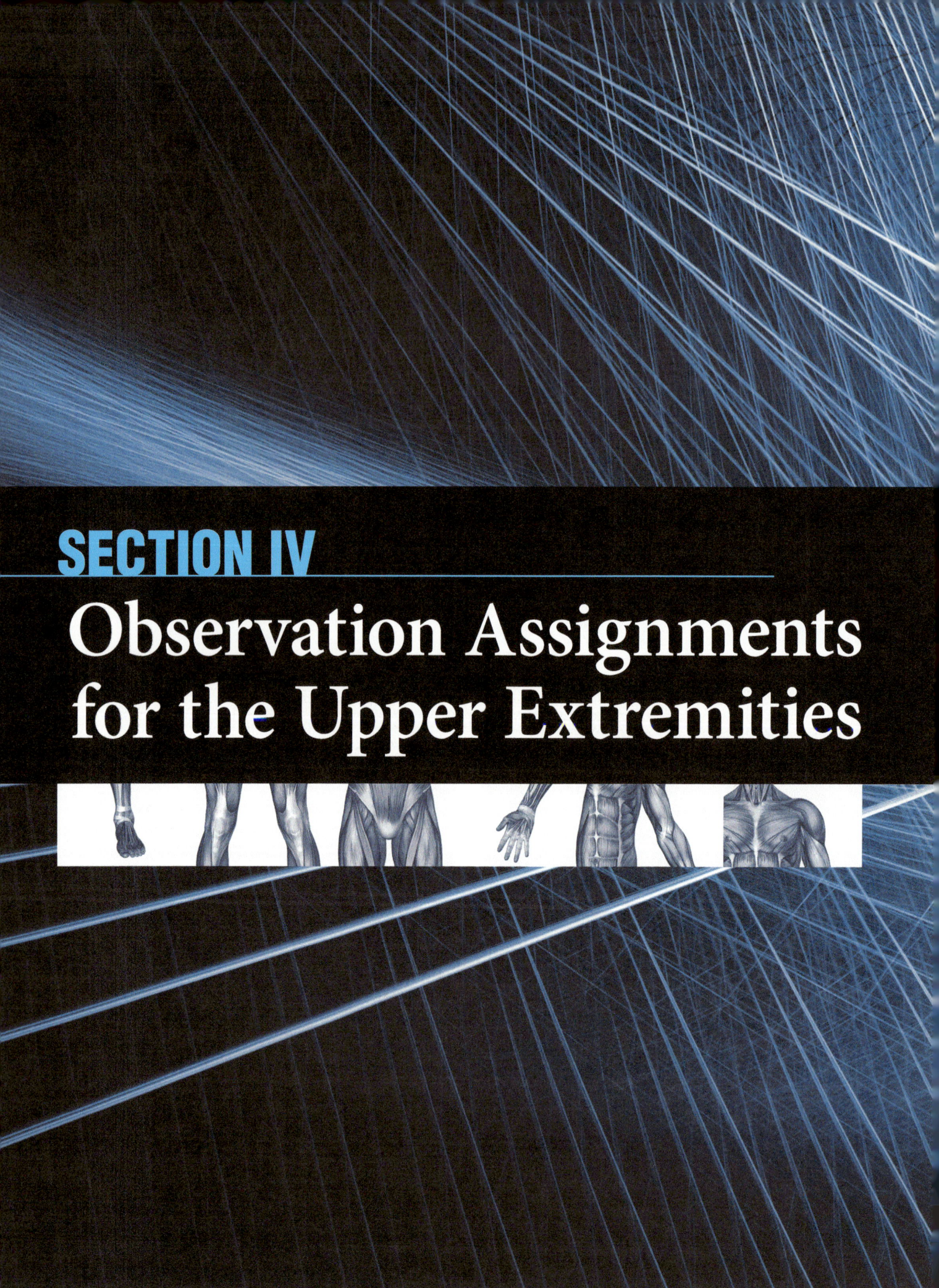

SECTION IV

Observation Assignments for the Upper Extremities

ASSIGNMENT 1—ORTHOPEDIC ROTATION

Perform an orthopedic rotation. Complete the following assignments based on that observation experience.

1. List all upper extremity injuries observed during observation experience, and also their mechanisms. Also, list if there was a previous injury of a similar nature.

_____

_____

_____

_____

_____

_____

_____

_____

_____

_____

_____

_____

2. Make a list of anything that could have prevented each of these injuries from occurring. Be specific.

_____

_____

_____

_____

_____

_____

_____

_____

_____

_____

_____

_____

3. List five treatments you observed, the injury being treated, and why that treatment was being given. What was the goal of each treatment?

_____

_____

_____

_____

_____

_____

_____

_____

_____

_____

_____

4. Do a mock upper extremity injury evaluation on a student with more experience or a certified professional. Write an injury report of the evaluation. Afterward, ask the student or professional to sign the evaluation to show that you have completed your evaluation in a systematic order.

_____

_____

_____

_____

_____

_____

_____

_____

_____

_____

_____

ASSIGNMENT 2—HAND AND WRIST

Observe a full evaluation of the hand and wrist and answer the following questions.

1. What was the mechanism of the injury?

_____

_____

_____

_____

_____

_____

_____

_____

_____

_____

2. Was there any noticeable swelling, deformity, or discoloration at the site of the injury? Did the patient hold the hand/wrist in a dependent position?

_____

_____

_____

_____

_____

_____

_____

_____

_____

_____

3. How was the patient's range of motion?

_____

_____

_____

_____

_____

_____

_____

_____

_____

_____

4. What muscles were tested, and what was the grade (0–5)?

_____

_____

_____

_____

_____

_____

_____

_____

_____

_____

_____

5. What ligamentous and special tests were performed? What was the result of each?

_____

_____

_____

_____

_____

_____

_____

_____

_____

_____

6. What neurological tests were performed? What was the result of each?

_____

_____

_____

_____

_____

_____

_____

_____

_____

_____

7. Comment on the evaluation. What do you think was performed correctly? What could have been done better? What did you learn from observing the evaluation?

_____

_____

_____

_____

_____

_____

_____

_____

_____

_____

_____

_____

ASSIGNMENT 3—ELBOW

Observe a full evaluation of the elbow and answer the following questions.

1. What was the mechanism of injury?

_____

_____

_____

_____

_____

_____

_____

_____

_____

_____

_____

2. Was there any noticeable swelling, deformity, or discoloration at the site of the injury? Did the patient guard or hold the injured elbow in a dependent position?

_____

_____

_____

_____

_____

_____

_____

_____

_____

_____

3. How was the patient's range of motion?

_____

_____

_____

_____

_____

_____

_____

_____

_____

_____

_____

_____

4. What muscles were tested, and what was the grade (0–5)?

_____

_____

_____

_____

_____

_____

_____

_____

_____

_____

_____

5. What ligamentous or special tests were performed? What was the result of each?

_____

_____

_____

_____

_____

_____

_____

_____

_____

_____

_____

_____

6. What neurological tests were performed? What was the result of each?

_____

_____

_____

_____

_____

_____

_____

_____

_____

_____

_____

7. Comment on the evaluation. What did you think was performed correctly? What could have been done better? What did you learn from observing the evaluation?

_____

_____

_____

_____

_____

_____

_____

_____

_____

_____

_____

_____

ASSIGNMENT 4—SHOULDER

Observe a full evaluation of the shoulder and answer the following questions.

1. What was the mechanism of the injury?

    _____

    _____

    _____

    _____

    _____

    _____

    _____

    _____

    _____

    _____

    _____

2. Was there any noticeable swelling, deformity, or discoloration at the site of the injury? Did the patient hold the injured arm in a dependent position?

    _____

    _____

    _____

    _____

    _____

    _____

    _____

    _____

    _____

    _____

    _____

    _____

3. How was the patient's range of motion?

_____

_____

_____

_____

_____

_____

_____

_____

_____

_____

4. What muscles were tested, and what was the grade (0–5)?

_____

_____

_____

_____

_____

_____

_____

_____

_____

_____

_____

5. What ligamentous or special tests were performed? What was the result of each?

_____

_____

_____

_____

_____

_____

_____

_____

_____

_____

6. What neurological tests were performed? What was the result of each?

_____

_____

_____

_____

_____

_____

_____

_____

_____

_____

_____

7. Comment on the evaluation. What do you think was performed correctly? What could have been done better? What did you learn from observing the evaluation?

_____

_____

_____

_____

_____

_____

_____

_____

_____

_____

Notes

Notes

Notes

UPPER EXTREMITY ACTIVITY MANUAL

Answers

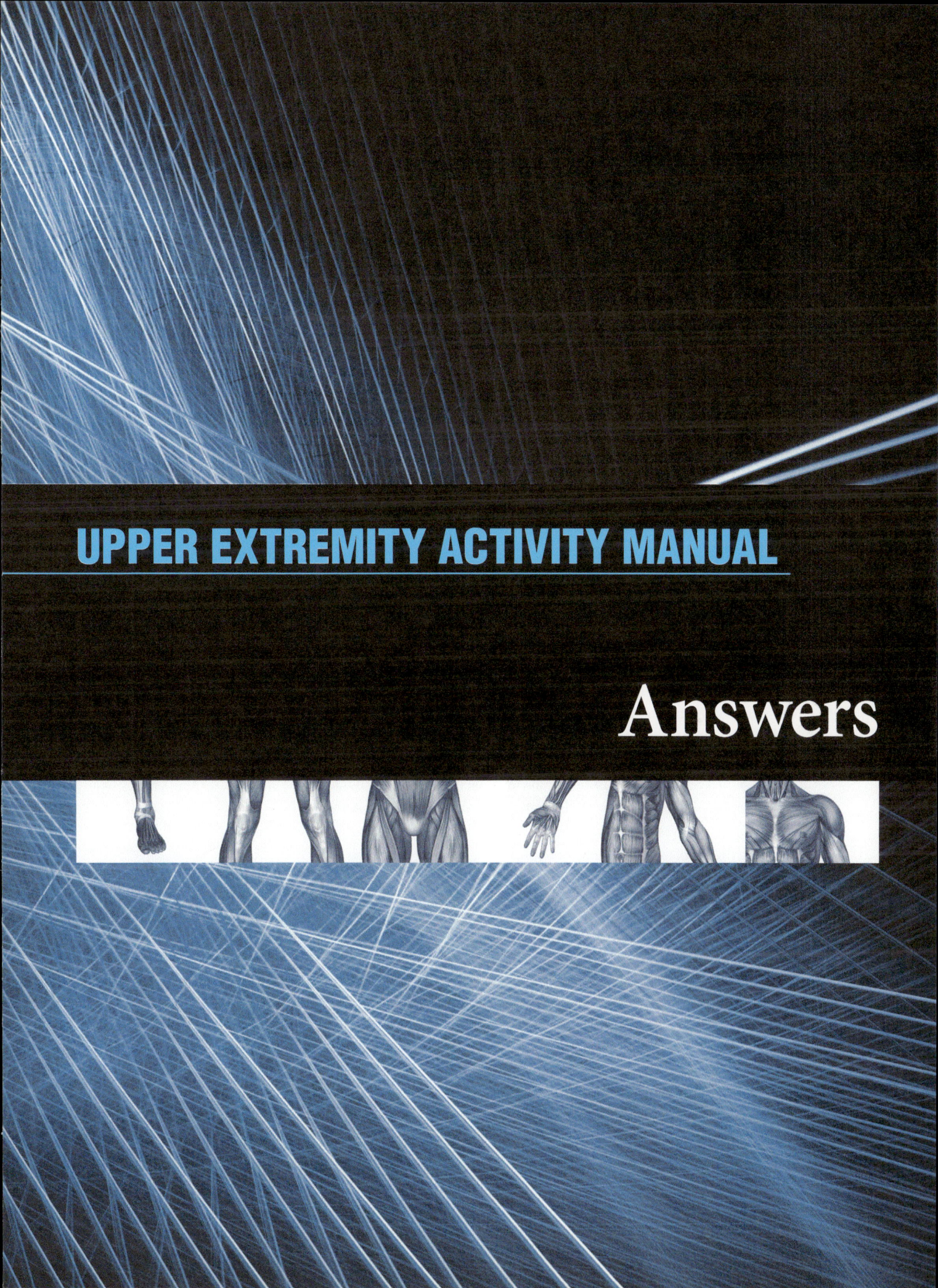

SCAVENGER HUNT ANSWERS FOR HAND AND WRIST

1. The triquetrum palpation is described as the last bone in the proximal row for the carpals.
2. The capitate is the largest of the carpal bones.
3. The two tendons that form the radial border of the anatomic snuff box are the extensor pollicis brevis and the abductor pollicis longus.
4. The mechanism of the injury mentioned is a fall on an outstretched hand.
5. The normal goniometric measurement for ulnar deviation is 30–35 degrees.
6. When testing the flexor digitorum superficialis, you should stabilize the MCP joint.
7. The muscles tested during the grip test are the opponens pollicis, oppenens digiti minimi, and lumbricales.
8. Clicking, pain, and excessive motion are positive results for the carpal glide test.
9. The Phalen's test should be held for one minute.
10. Murphy's sign occurs when the third metacarpal is even with the second and fourth.

RELATED HAND AND WRIST QUESTIONS

1. A benign mass (tumor) usually seen on the dorsal side of the wrist is referred to as a ganglion cyst.
2. A gamekeeper's injury results in pathology to the ulnar collateral ligament of the thumb.
3. Mallet finger is an avulsion of the extensor tendon with inability to extend at the DIP joint, whereas jersey finger is avulsion of the flexor digitorum profundis with inability to flex at the DIP joint.
4. The most commonly fractured bone in the hand is the scaphoid.
5. The most commonly dislocated bone in the wrist is the lunate.
6. When measuring ulnar deviation the fulcrum is placed on the capitate.
7. A disease that results in necrosis of the lunate bone due to a loss of blood supply is called kienbock's disease.
8. Blood trapped under the fingernail is referred to as a subungual hematoma.
9. The two major nerves that innervate the wrist and hand are the ulnar and median nerves.
10. Bringing the thumb and little finger together is an example of opposition.
11. A fracture of the first metacarpal that extends into the articular surface is called a bennet's fracture.
12. Fractures of the fifth metacarpal are termed boxer fractures.
13. When splinting a mallet finger, the distal interphalangeal (DIP) joint should be in extension.
14. There are eight carpal bones in the hand.
15. Movement of the hand toward the radial side is termed radial deviation.

16.

MUSCLE	ORIGIN	INSERTION	ACTION	INNERVATION
Flexor digitorum profundis	Upper 3/4 of ulna, medial epicondyle and coronoid process of the ulna	Distal phalanx of fingers 2–5	Finger flexion PIP and DIP and wrist flexion	Median and ulnar
Flexor digitorum superficialis	Common flexor tendon, coronoid process, and radius	Sides of middle phalanx of fingers 2–5	Finger flexion PIP and DIP and wrist flexion	Median
Extensor pollicis longus	Mid-posterior surface of ulna	Base of distal phalanx	Thumb extension	Radial
Abductor pollicis longus	Posterior surface of radius and middle ulna	Base of fifth metacarpal	Thumb abduction	Radial
Adductor pollicis	Capitate, base of second metacarpal, palmar surface third metacarpal	Base of proximal phalanx of thumb	Thumb adduction	Ulnar

17.

MOTION	MOVABLE ARM	STATIONARY ARM	FULCRUM	NORMAL RANGE OF MOTION
Wrist flexion	Fifth metacarpal	Ulna	Triquetrum	90 degrees
Wrist extension	Fifth metacarpal	Ulna	Triquetrum	70 degrees
Ulnar deviation	Third metacarpal	Midline forearm	Capitate	30 degrees
Radial deviation	Third metacarpal	Midline forearm	Capitate	20 degrees

PALPATION LESSON

You are teaching a lab class on hand and wrist palpation. For the following palpations, explain how you would locate each.

PALPATION	LOCATION EXPLANATION
1. Lister's tubercle	Follow the radius in a distal direction to the radial styloid process. Move toward the middle of the hand. Lister's tubercle is about a 1/3 of the way over, even with the third metacarpal.
2. Triquetrum	Start with the ulnar styloid process, and move distally, add some radial deviation and the triquetrum will pop under your thumb when the wrist is fully radially deviated.
3. TFCC	Palpate distal from the ulnar styloid on the medial side. The TFCC sits between the head of the fifth metacarpal and the ulna.
4. Extensor pollicis longus	Have the patient go into the thumbs up position to form the anatomic snuff box. The Extensor pollicis longus is the long tendon on the ulnar border of the anatomical snuff box.
5. Palmaris longus	The palmaris longus tendon is located in the middle of the ventral side of the forearm and is accentuated by having the patient flex their wrist and opposing the thumb and finger.
6. Hypothenar eminence	Follow the fifth phalange proximally. The fleshy part of the hand on the ulnar side is the hypothenar eminence.
7. Pisiform	The pisiform is the pebble-like projection just distal to the ulna on the palmar side. It feels like a very superficial pebble underneath your finger.
8. Radial artery	The radial artery is on the palmar surface and just medial from the radial styloid process.
9. Ulnar collateral ligament of the thumb	Palpate all along the ulnar side of the metacarpal phalange joint. The ulnar collateral ligament attaches distally at the proximal phalanx.

 # SCAVENGER HUNT ANSWERS FOR ELBOW

1. The radial head can be made more prominent by asking the client to pronate and supinate his or her forearm.
2. When the palm of the hand is placed on the medial epicondyle, the index finger points to the flexor carpi radialis.
3. The normal range of motion for forearm pronation is 90–96 degrees.
4. The forearm is placed in the neutral position when testing the brachioradialis.
5. The elbow is flexed 20–30 degrees when performing valgus or varus stress testing.
6. Tinel's sign is completed for the ulnar nerve.
7. The ulnar nerve is found in the groove posterior to the medial epicondyle.
8. The triceps is the only muscle mentioned that is responsible for elbow extension.
9. The mechanisms mentioned are throwing and attempting to tackle a passing player.
10. The structure palpated during the tennis elbow test is the lateral epicondyle.

RELATED ELBOW QUESTIONS

1. The normal carrying angle of the elbow in women is between 10 and 15 degrees.
2. The wrist extensor group of muscles originates on the lateral epicondyle of the humerus.
3. The primary resistance to a valgus force placed on the elbow is the medial collateral ligament.
4. The olecranon bursa is the most frequently injured bursa in the elbow.
5. Pitcher's elbow and little league elbow affect the medial epicondyle of the humerus.
6. A 3 out of 5 grade on a triceps manual muscle test means that the elbow moves against gravity in full range of motion but cannot hold against resistance.
7. When a client is diagnosed with a grade II MCL sprain of the elbow, their signs and symptoms likely include pain, swelling, laxity, pain on valgus stress, and a strength deficit.
8. The elbow joint is made of three bones.
9.

MUSCLE	ORIGIN	INSERTION	ACTION	INNERVATION
Biceps brachii (long head)	Supraglenoid tubercle of scapula	Radial tuberosity of radius	Flexion elbow and arm and supination of forearm	Musculocutaneous
Triceps brachii (long head)	Infraglenoid tubercle of scapula	Olecranon process of ulna	Extension of elbow and arm	Radial
Brachialis	Anterior surface of distal half of humerus	Coronoid process, ulnar tuberosity of ulna	Flexion	Musculocutaneous
Pronator teres	Medial epicondyle of humerus/coronoid process of ulna	Lateral surface of radius at midpoint	Forearm pronation	Median
Flexor carpi radialis	Medial epicondyle of humerus	Base of second and third metacarpals	Wrist flexion/radial deviation	Median

ANSWERS

10.

MOTION	MOVABLE ARM	STATIONARY ARM	FULCRUM	NORMAL RANGE OF MOTION
Elbow flexion	Radius	Lateral humerus	Lateral epicondyle	140–150 degrees
Elbow extension	Radius	Lateral humerus	Lateral epicondyle	0 degrees
Pronation	Straight up	Perpendicular to floor	MCP joint of third phalange	90–96 degrees
Supination	Straight up	Perpendicular to floor	MCP joint of third phalange	81–93 degrees

PALPATION LESSON

You are teaching a lab class on elbow palpation. For the following palpations, explain how you would locate each.

PALPATION	LOCATION EXPLANATION
1. Olecranon	This is the rounded part of the elbow located on the posterior surface. Start at the anterior cubital fossa and palpate the rounded posterior surface (which is the olecranon).
2. Ulnar nerve	Start at the medial epicondyle and slide posterior into the groove. In this groove is the ulnar nerve.
3. Pronator teres	Place the palm of your hand on the medial epicondyle. The thumb is over the pronator teres.
4. Radial head	Palpate the lateral epicondyle of the humerus and then move inferiorly and have the patient pronate and supinate their forearm, the radial head will become more prominent.
5. Brachioradialis	Have the patient do an isometric hammer type bicep curl and the muscle belly becomes prominent on the top portion of the forearm.
6. Lateral epicondyle	The lateral epicondyle is located on the lateral side at the same level as the medial epicondyle. It is a rounded projection on the lateral aspect of the elbow.
7. Medial collateral ligament	Injury to the medial collateral ligament may produce pain from the medial epicondyle to the medial side of the proximal ulna.
8. Brachial artery	The artery can be found by following the bicep muscle to its midpoint and moving medially.

SCAVENGER HUNT ANSWERS FOR SHOULDER

1. External rotation of the humerus will make the lesser tuberosity more prominent.
2. A SLAP lesion refers to a superior labrum tear from anterior to posterior.
3. Impingement syndrome affects the subscapularis and supraspinatus muscles.
4. If an athlete sustained an AC joint sprain, it would be important to palpate the AC joint, Clavicle, and SC joint. To determine ligament stability, the examiner could complete the AC joint stress test, AC joint distraction test, and the piano key sign.
5. A stinger is a brachial plexus injury resulting in numbness and tingling down the arm.
6. Bicep tendonitis causes pain in the bicipital groove.
7. The majority of clavicle fractures occur where the concave meets the convex portion of the clavicle.
8. A goniometric measurement for shoulder flexion is approximately 160–180 degrees.
9. GIRD stands for glenohumeral internal rotation deficiency.
10. The special tests that could be used to diagnose glenohumeral joint instability include apprehension, Jobe relocation, posterior apprehension, sulcus, anterior drawer, posterior drawer, load/shift, and Feagin.

RELATED SHOULDER QUESTIONS

1. The shoulder girdle is made up of the clavicle, scapula, and humerus.
2. The lateral aspect of the upper arm is the most common site for Myositis ossificans in the shoulder.
3. The spine of the scapula is at the same level as the T3 spinous process.
4. The inferior angle of the scapula is at the same level as the seventh rib.
5. If you suspect an athlete is suffering from impingement syndrome, you would likely perform the Crossover, Neer, and Hawkins-Kennedy special tests.
6. To differentiate the injured structure when performing an AC joint distraction test, you should note if the step-off deformity is below the acromion, indicating a glenohumeral pathology.
7. The piano key sign will be positive if an athlete is suffering from a second or third degree AC joint separation.
8. When performing the drop arm test an inability to slowly lower the arm is indicative of a rotator cuff tear.
9. A grade of 4 on a manual muscle test is indicative of movement against gravity through a full range of motion, and holds moderate but not full resistance.
10. Erb's point is located 2–3 cm above the convex portion of the clavicle, the area where the brachial plexus is most superficial.

11.

MUSCLE	ORIGIN	INSERTION	ACTION	INNERVATION
Deltoid (anterior)	Lateral 1/3 of clavicle, anterior superior surface	Deltoid tuberosity of humerus	Abduction, flexion and medial rotation	Axillary
Pectoralis major (sternal)	Sternum, ribs 2–7	Lateral lip of bicipital groove	Horizontal adduction	Lateral and medial pectoral nerve
Teres minor	Axillary border of scapula	Greater tubercle of humerus	External rotation	Axillary
Levator scapulae	C1–C4 vertebrae	Scapula (vertebral border)	Scapular elevation	Third to fourth cervical nerves, dorsal scapular nerve
Latissimus dorsi	Spinous process T7–L5, sacrum, iliac crest, lower three ribs	Medial lip of bicipital groove	Internal rotation, extension and adduction	Thoracodorsal
Rhomboid minor	C7–T1 spinous process	Spine of scapula	Scapula retraction and downward rotation	Dorsal scapular
Supraspinatus	Supraspinatus fossa, scapula	Greater tubercle of humerus	Abduction	Suprascapular

12.

MOTION	MOVABLE ARM	STATIONARY ARM	FULCRUM	NORMAL RANGE OF MOTION
Shoulder extension	Lateral humerus	Lateral torso parallel to midline	Acromium	50–60 degrees
Shoulder flexion	Lateral humerus	Lateral torso parallel to midline	Acromium	160–180 degrees
Shoulder internal rotation	Ulnar styloid process	Perpendicular to the floor	Olecranon	60–70 degrees
Shoulder external rotation	Ulnar styloid process	Perpendicular to the floor	Olecranon	80–90 degrees

PALPATION LESSON

You are teaching a lab class on shoulder palpation. For the following palpations, explain how you would locate each.

PALPATION	LOCATION EXPLANATION
1. AC joint	Follow the clavicle out to the acromioclavicular joint, also known as the AC joint. This is where the acromion and the clavicle articulate.
2. Spine of scapula	Start at the acromion and palpate the posterior shoulder. The spine of the scapula is located on the proximal one-third of the scapula and is the most prominent portion of the scapula that can be felt.
3. Bicipital groove	Locate the lesser and greater tuberosity of the humerus, the divot located between the two is the bicipital groove. Internal and external rotation will facilitate this palpation.
4. Deltoid tuberosity	Start at the acromion follow the deltoid muscle down to where it dips and attaches to the humerus, this is the deltoid tuberosity.
5. Subacromial bursa	Place the arm into slight extension and the subacromial bursa is right under the acromion.
6. Lateral border of the scapula	Start at the spine of the scapula, palpate lateral, and deeper underneath the muscles, If not distinguishable in a neutral position, have the patient place the dorsum of the wrist on the PSIS, this should facilitate palpation of the lateral border of the scapula.
7. Sternal notch	From the sternoclavicular joint move medial. The divot felt is the sternal notch.
8. Lesser tuberosity of humerus	Start at the easier to find greater tuberosity and externally rotate the shoulder, the lesser tuberosity will become more prominent.

HAND AND WRIST

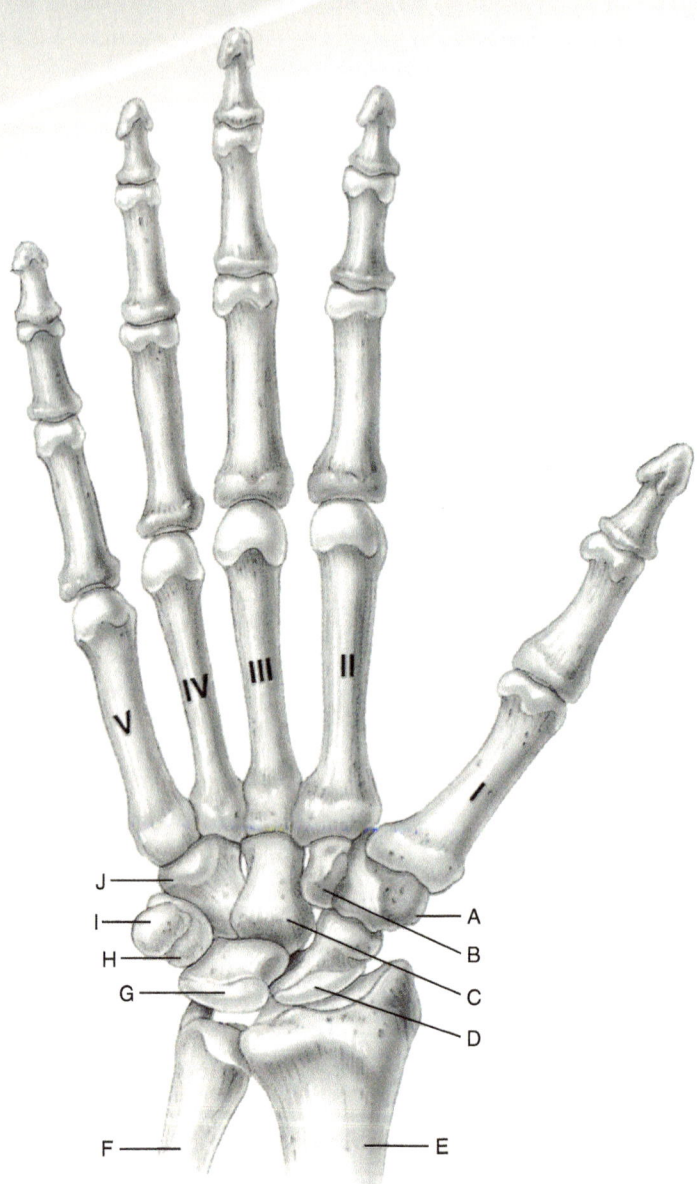

FIGURE 1-1

A. Trapezium
B. Trapezoid
C. Capitate
D. Scaphoid
E. Radius

F. Ulna
G. Lunate
H. Triquetrium
I. Pisiform
J. Hamate

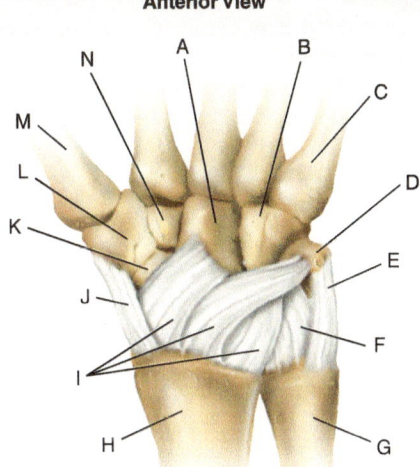

Anterior View

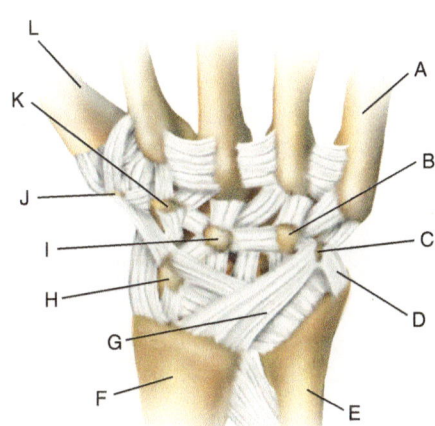

Posterior View

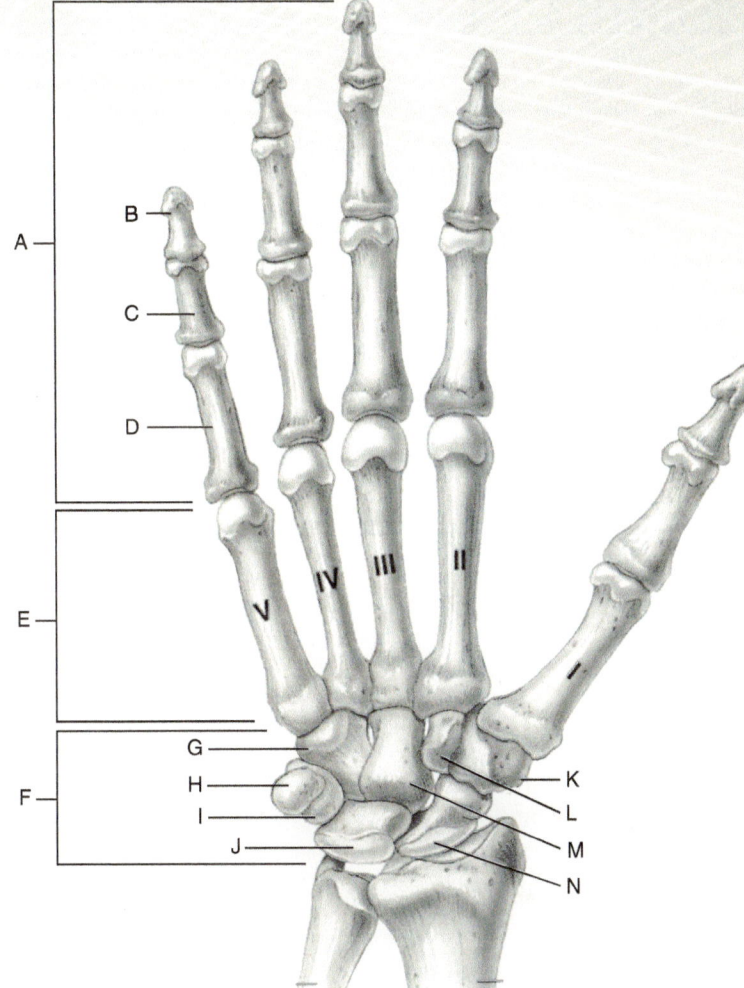

FIGURE 1-2

Anterior View

A. Capitate
B. Hamate
C. Fifth metacarpal
D. Pisiform
E. Ulnar collateral ligament
F. Palmar ulnocarpal ligament
G. Ulna
H. Radius

I. Palmar radiocarpal ligament
J. Radial collateral ligament
K. Scaphoid
L. Trapezium
M. First metacarpal
N. Trapezoid

Posterior View

A. Fifth metacarpal
B. Hamate
C. Triquetrium
D. Ulnar collateral ligament
E. Ulna
F. Radius

G. Dorsal radiocarpal ligament
H. Scaphoid
I. Capitate
J. Trapezium
K. Trapezoid
L. First metacarpal

FIGURE 1-3
A. Phalanges
B. Distal phalanx
C. Middle phalanx
D. Proximal phalanx
E. Metacarpals
F. Carpals
G. Hamate

H. Pisiform
I. Triquetrium
J. Lunate
K. Trapezium
L. Trapezoid
M. Capitate
N. Scaphoid

ELBOW

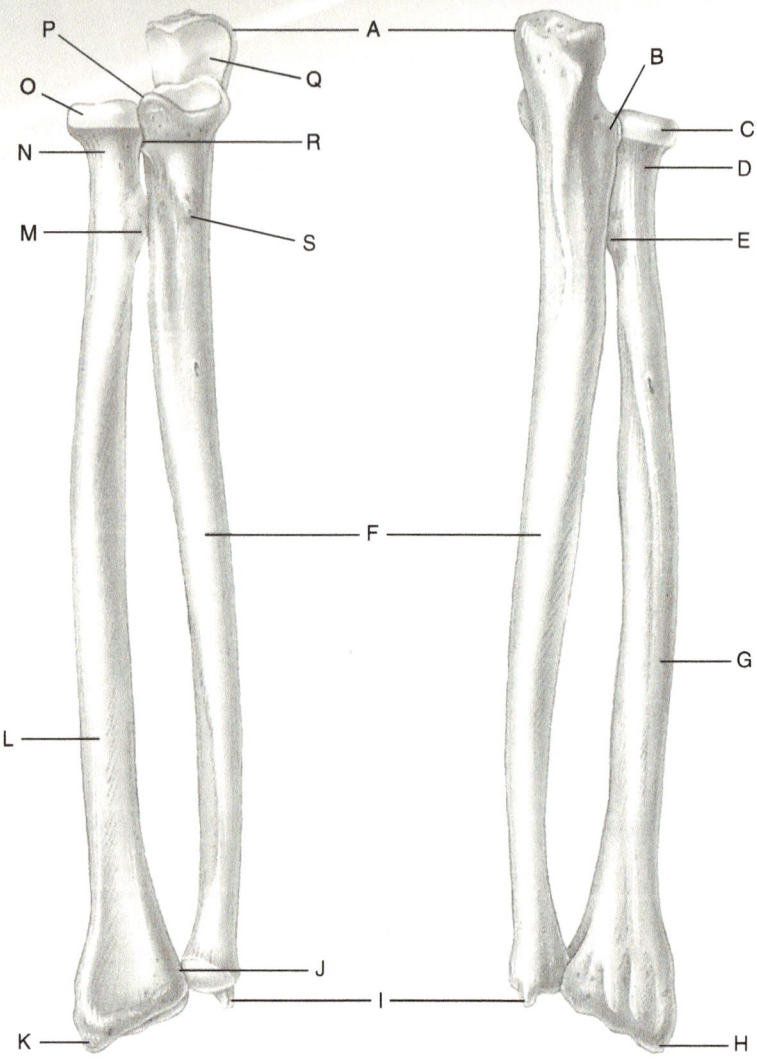

Anterior View   **Posterior View**

FIGURE 2-1

A. Oleacranon
B. Coronoid process
C. Head of radius
D. Neck of radius
E. Radial tuberosity
F. Ulna
G. Radius [posterior side]
H. Styloid process of radius [posterior]
I. Styloid process of ulna
J. Distal radioulnar joint
K. Styloid process of radius [anterior]

L. Radius [anterior]
M. Radial tuberosity [anterior]
N. Neck of radius [anterior]
O. Head of radius [anterior]
P. Radial notch
Q. Trochlear notch
R. Proximal radioulnar joint
S. Ulnar tuberosity

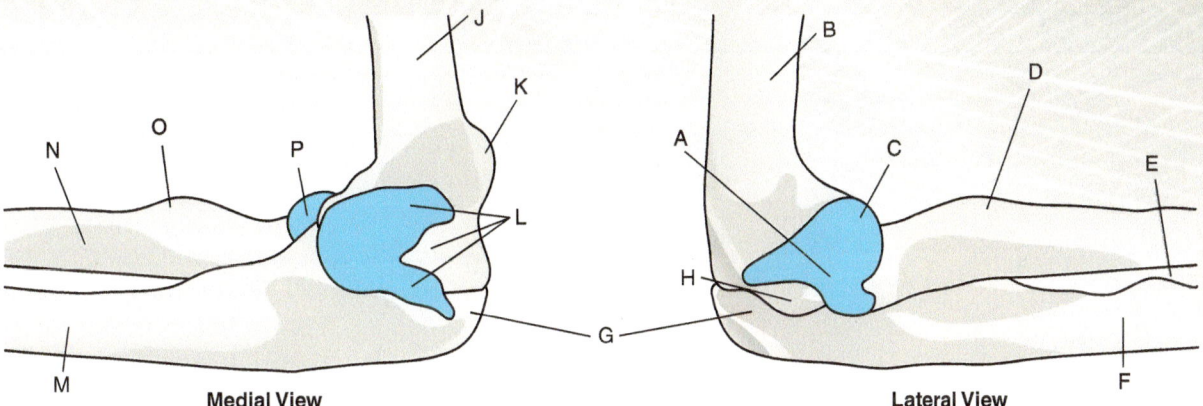

Medial View   **Lateral View**

FIGURE 2-2

Lateral View
A. Radial collateral ligament
B. Humerus
C. Annular ligament
D. Radial tuberosity
E. Antebrachial interosseous membrane
F. Ulna
G. Oleacranon of ulna [points to both]
H. Capitulum
I. Radial collateral ligament

Medial View
J. Humerus
K. Medial epicondyle
L. Ulnar collateral ligaments
M. Ulna
N. Radius
O. Radial tuberosity
P. Annular ligament

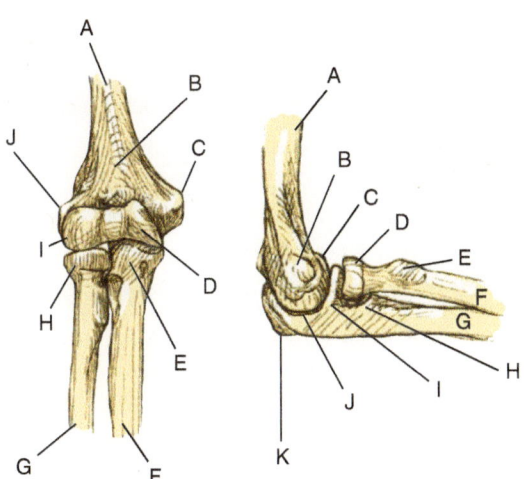

Anterior   **Lateral**

FIGURE 2-3

Anterior
A. Humerus
B. Coronoid fossa
C. Medial epicondyle
D. Trochlea
E. Ulnar coronoid epicondyle
F. Ulna
G. Radius
H. Radial head
I. Capitulum (capitellum)
J. Lateral epicondyle
K. Oleacranon process

Lateral
A. Humerus
B. Lateral epicondyle
C. Capitulum
D. Head
E. Tuberosity
F. Radius
G. Ulna
H. Radial notch of ulna
I. Coronoid process
J. Trochlear notch

SHOULDER

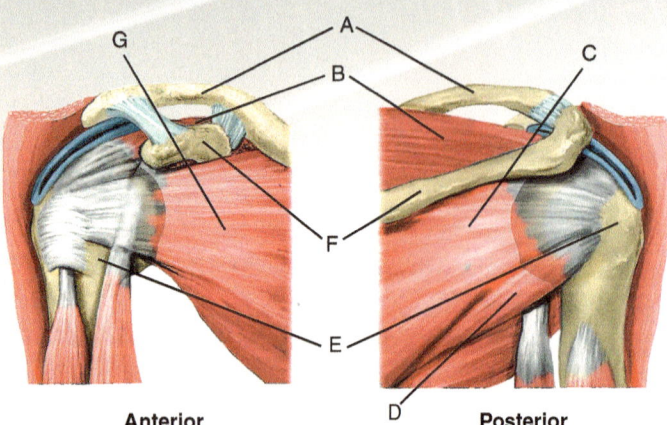

Anterior   **Posterior**

FIGURE 3-1

A. Clavicle
B. Supraspinatus
C. Infraspinatus
D. Teres minor

E. Humerus
F. Scapula
G. Subscapularis

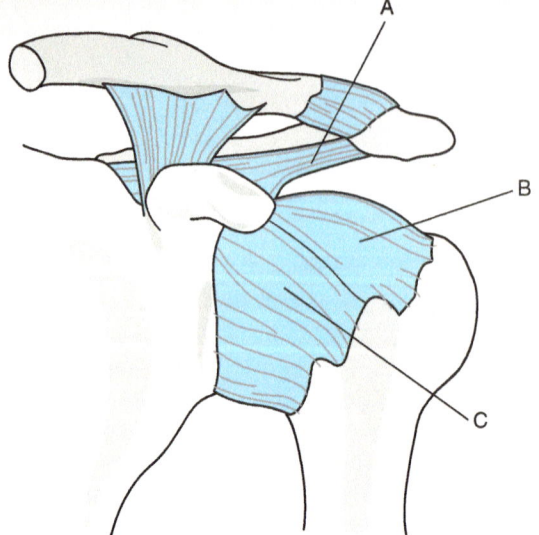

FIGURE 3-2

A. Coracoacromial ligament
B. Coracohumeral ligament
C. Glenohumeral ligament

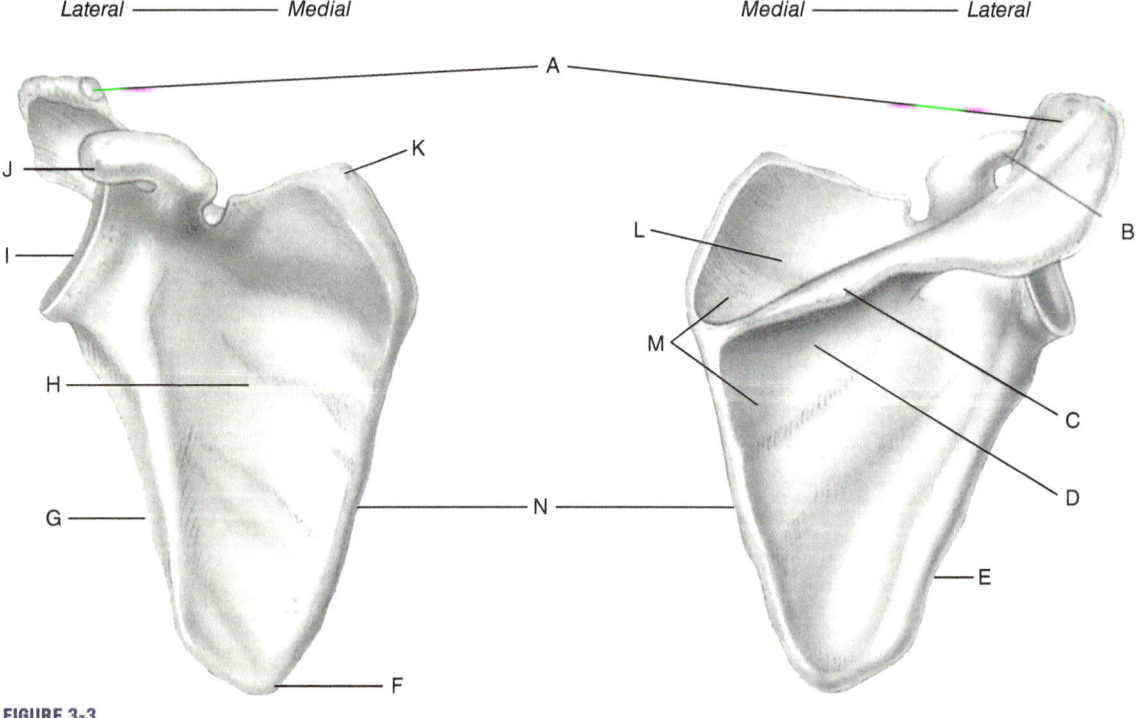

Lateral ——— Medial   *Medial ——— Lateral*

FIGURE 3-3

A. Acromion process
B. Coracoid process
C. Spinous process
D. Intraspinous fossa
E. Axillary border

F. Inferior angle
G. Axillary border
H. Subscapular fossa
I. Glenoid fossa
J. Coracoid process

K. Superior angle
L. Supraspinous fossa
M. Body
N. Vertebral border

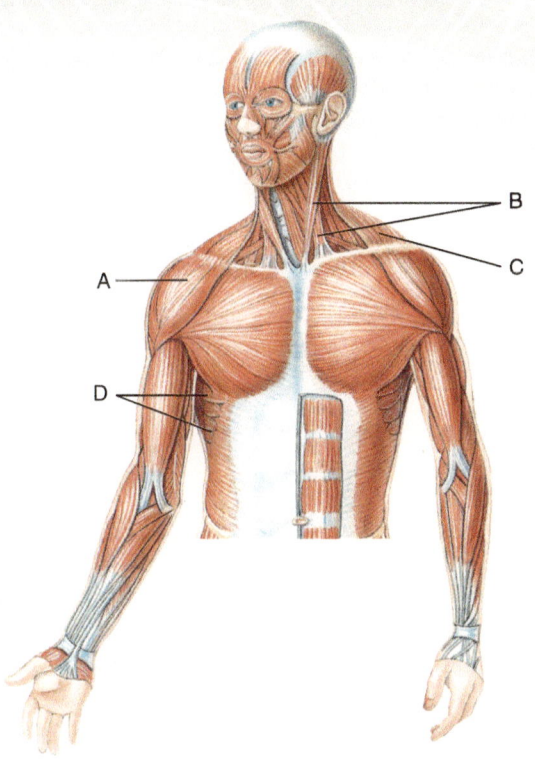

FIGURE 3-4
A. Deltoid
B. Sternocleidomastoid
C. Trapezius
D. Serratus anterior

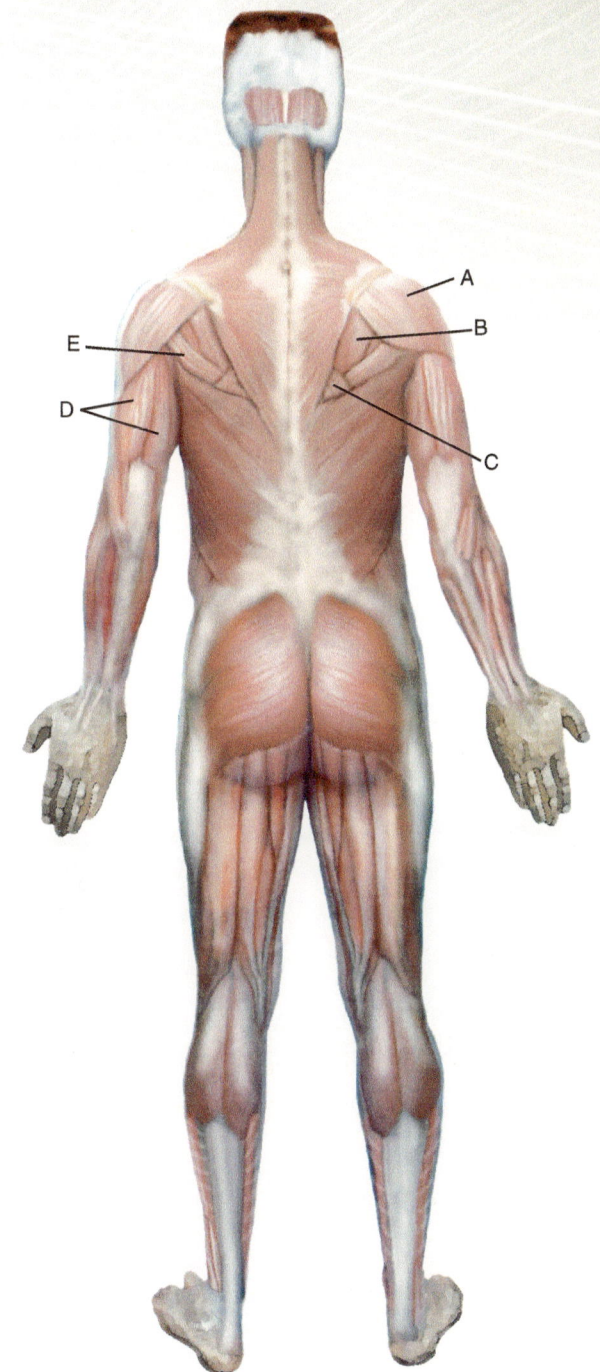

FIGURE 3-5
A. Deltoid
B. Infraspinatus
C. Rhomboideus major
D. Triceps brachii
E. Teres major

Index

Minimum System Requirements

- Microsoft Windows XP w/SP 2, Windows Vista w/ SP 1, Windows 7
- Mac OS X 10.4, 10.5, or 10.6
- Processor: Minimum required by Operating System
- Memory: Minimum required by Operating System
- Screen resolution: 1024 × 768 pixels
- CD-ROM drive
- Sound card & listening device required for audio features
- Flash Player 10. The Adobe Flash Player is free, and can be downloaded from http://www.adobe.com/products/flashplayer/

Windows Setup Instructions

1. Insert disc into CD-ROM drive. The software program should start automatically. If it does not, go to step 2.
2. From My Computer, double-click the icon for the CD drive.
3. Double-click the *InjuryEval.exe* file to start the program.

Mac Setup Instructions

1. Insert disc into CD-ROM drive.
2. Once the disc icon appears on your desktop, double click on it to open it.
3. Double-click the *Injury Evaluation* file to start the program.

Technical Support

Telephone: 1-800-648-7450

8:30 A.M.–6:30 P.M. Eastern Time

E-mail: delmar.help@cengage.com

3.2 Cengage Learning reserves the right at any time to withdraw from the Licensed Content any item or part of an item for which it no longer retains the right to publish, or which it has reasonable grounds to believe infringes copyright or is defamatory, unlawful, or otherwise objectionable.

4.0 PROTECTION AND SECURITY

4.1 The End User shall use its best efforts and take all reasonable steps to safeguard its copy of the Licensed Content to ensure that no unauthorized reproduction, publication, disclosure, modification, or distribution of the Licensed Content, in whole or in part, is made. To the extent that the End User becomes aware of any such unauthorized use of the Licensed Content, the End User shall immediately notify Cengage Learning. Notification of such violations may be made by sending an e-mail to infringement@cengage.com.

5.0 MISUSE OF THE LICENSED PRODUCT

5.1 In the event that the End User uses the Licensed Content in violation of this Agreement, Cengage Learning shall have the option of electing liquidated damages, which shall include all profits generated by the End User's use of the Licensed Content plus interest computed at the maximum rate permitted by law and all legal fees and other expenses incurred by Cengage Learning in enforcing its rights, plus penalties.

6.0 FEDERAL GOVERNMENT CLIENTS

6.1 Except as expressly authorized by Cengage Learning, Federal Government clients obtain only the rights specified in this Agreement and no other rights. The Government acknowledges that (i) all software and related documentation incorporated in the Licensed Content is existing commercial computer software within the meaning of FAR 27.405(b)(2); and (2) all other data delivered in whatever form, is limited rights data within the meaning of FAR 27.401. The restrictions in this section are acceptable as consistent with the Government's need for software and other data under this Agreement.

7.0 DISCLAIMER OF WARRANTIES AND LIABILITIES

7.1 Although Cengage Learning believes the Licensed Content to be reliable, Cengage Learning does not guarantee or warrant (i) any information or materials contained in or produced by the Licensed Content, (ii) the accuracy, completeness or reliability of the Licensed Content, or (iii) that the Licensed Content is free from errors or other material defects. THE LICENSED PRODUCT IS PROVIDED "AS IS," WITHOUT ANY WARRANTY OF ANY KIND AND CENGAGE LEARNING DISCLAIMS ANY AND ALL WARRANTIES, EXPRESSED OR IMPLIED, INCLUDING, WITHOUT LIMITATION, WARRANTIES OF MERCHANTABILITY OR FITNESS FOR A PARTICULAR PURPOSE. IN NO EVENT SHALL CENGAGE LEARNING BE LIABLE FOR: INDIRECT, SPECIAL, PUNITIVE OR CONSEQUENTIAL DAMAGES INCLUDING FOR LOST PROFITS, LOST DATA, OR OTHERWISE. IN NO EVENT SHALL CENGAGE LEARNING'S AGGREGATE LIABILITY HEREUNDER, WHETHER ARISING IN CONTRACT, TORT, STRICT LIABILITY OR OTHERWISE, EXCEED THE AMOUNT OF FEES PAID BY THE END USER HEREUNDER FOR THE LICENSE OF THE LICENSED CONTENT.

8.0 GENERAL

8.1 Entire Agreement. This Agreement shall constitute the entire Agreement between the Parties and supercedes all prior Agreements and understandings oral or written relating to the subject matter hereof.

8.2 Enhancements/Modifications of Licensed Content. From time to time, and in Cengage Learning's sole discretion, Cengage Learning may advise the End User of updates, upgrades, enhancements and/or improvements to the Licensed Content, and may permit the End User to access and use, subject to the terms and conditions of this Agreement, such modifications, upon payment of prices as may be established by Cengage Learning.

8.3 No Export. The End User shall use the Licensed Content solely in the United States and shall not transfer or export, directly or indirectly, the Licensed Content outside the United States.

8.4 Severability. If any provision of this Agreement is invalid, illegal, or unenforceable under any applicable statute or rule of law, the provision shall be deemed omitted to the extent that it is invalid, illegal, or unenforceable. In such a case, the remainder of the Agreement shall be construed in a manner as to give greatest effect to the original intention of the parties hereto.

8.5 Waiver. The waiver of any right or failure of either party to exercise in any respect any right provided in this Agreement in any instance shall not be deemed to be a waiver of such right in the future or a waiver of any other right under this Agreement.

8.6 Choice of Law/Venue. This Agreement shall be interpreted, construed, and governed by and in accordance with the laws of the State of New York, applicable to contracts executed and to be wholly preformed therein, without regard to its principles governing conflicts of law. Each party agrees that any proceeding arising out of or relating to this Agreement or the breach or threatened breach of this Agreement may be commenced and prosecuted in a court in the State and County of New York. Each party consents and submits to the nonexclusive personal jurisdiction of any court in the State and County of New York in respect of any such proceeding.

8.7 Acknowledgment. By opening this package and/or by accessing the Licensed Content on this Web site, THE END USER ACKNOWLEDGES THAT IT HAS READ THIS AGREEMENT, UNDERSTANDS IT, AND AGREES TO BE BOUND BY ITS TERMS AND CONDITIONS. IF YOU DO NOT ACCEPT THESE TERMS AND CONDITIONS, YOU MUST NOT ACCESS THE LICENSED CONTENT AND RETURN THE LICENSED PRODUCT TO CENGAGE LEARNING (WITHIN 30 CALENDAR DAYS OF THE END USER'S PURCHASE) WITH PROOF OF PAYMENT ACCEPTABLE TO CENGAGE LEARNING, FOR A CREDIT OR A REFUND. Should the End User have any questions/comments regarding this Agreement, please contact Cengage Learning at Delmar.help@cengage.com.